Step
Inno
Presbyopia Management

Editors

Ashok Garg
MS PhD FIAO(Bel) FRSM
FAIMS ADM FICA
International and National
Gold Medalist
Medical Director
Garg Eye Institute and
Research Centre
235-Model Town
Dabra Chowk
Hisar-125005
India

Guillermo Avalos Urzua
MD
Chief Ophthalmic Deptt.
Sagrado, Corazon Hospital
Medical Director
Avalos Ophthalmic
Institute and
Ophthalmic Laser Clinic
Terranova No. 676-101
Col. Providencia
Guadalajara, Jal, Mexico
CP 44630

Dimitrii Dementiev
MD
Chief and Medical Director
Blue Eye Centro di
Michrochirurgia Oculare
Eye Clinic, Arese 20020 (MI)
Via Campo Gallo 21/10
Milan, Italy

Roberto Pinelli
MD
Scientific Director
Instituto Laser
Microchirurgia Oculare
Crystal Palace
Via Cefalonia 70
Brescia-25124, Italy

***Foreword:* Marguerite B McDonald**

JAYPEE BROTHERS
MEDICAL PUBLISHERS (P) LTD
New Delhi

Published by

Jitendar P Vij
Jaypee Brothers Medical Publishers (P) Ltd
EMCA House, 23/23B Ansari Road, Daryaganj
New Delhi 110 002, India
Phones: +91-11-23272143, +91-11-23272703, +91-11-23282021, +91-11-23245672
Fax: +91-11-23276490, +91-11-23245683
e-mail: jaypee@jaypeebrothers.com
Visit our website: www.jaypeebrothers.com

Branches

- 202 Batavia Chambers, 8 Kumara Krupa Road
Kumara Park East, **Bangalore** 560 001
Phones: +91-80-22285971, +91-80-22382956, +91-80-30614073
Tele Fax : +91-80-22281761 e-mail: jaypeebc@bgl.vsnl.net.in
- 282 IIIrd Floor, Khaleel Shirazi Estate, Fountain Plaza
Pantheon Road, **Chennai** 600 008
Phones: +91-44-28262665, +91-44-28269897
Fax: +91-44-28262331 e-mail: jpchen@eth.net
- 4-2-1067/1-3, 1st Floor, Balaji Building, Ramkote Cross Road
Hyderabad 500 095, Phones: +91-40-55610020, +91-40-24758498
Fax: +91-40-24758499 e-mail: jpmedpub@rediffmail.com
- 1A Indian Mirror Street, Wellington Square
Kolkata 700 013, Phones: +91-33-22456075, +91-33-22451926
Fax: +91-33-2245607 e-mail: jpbcal@cal.vsnl.net.in
- 106 Amit Industrial Estate, 61 Dr SS Rao Road
Near MGM Hospital, Parel, **Mumbai** 400 012
Phones: +91-22-24124863, +91-22-24104532, +91-22-30926896
Fax: +91-22-24160828 e-mail: jpmedpub@bom7.vsnl.net.in
- "KAMALPUSHPA" 38, Reshimbag
Opp. Mohota Science College, Umred Road, **Nagpur** 440 009 (MS)
Phone: +91-712-3945220, e-mail: jpnagpur@rediffmail.com

Step by Step Innovations in Presbyopia Management

First Edition : **2006**

ISBN 81-8061-647-9

Typeset at JPBMP typesetting unit

Printed at Paras Offset Pvt. Ltd., New Delhi

Dedicated to

- My respected Param Pujya Guru Sant Gurmeet Ram Rahim Singh Ji for his blessings and motivation.
- My respected parents, teachers, my wife Dr Aruna Garg, son Abhishek and daughter Anshul for their constant support and patience during all these days of hard work.
- My dear friend Dr Amar Agarwal, a renowned International Ophthalmologist, for his constant support, guidance and expertise.

— Ashok Garg

- In loving memory of my father whom's example lay the footsteps for me to follow.
- To my wife with love and to my children may they achieve professional and personal fulfillment.

— Guillermo Avalos Urzua

- My friend and my teacher in Ophthalmology Prof. Viktor Zuev MD.

— Dimitrii Dementiev

- I dedicate this book to India's talented ophthalmologists, in the fervent hope that they may become increasingly devoted to refractive surgery.

— Roberto Pinelli

Contributors

Amar Agarwal MS FRCS FRC Ophth
Consultant
Dr Agarwal's Eye Hospital
19, Cathedral Road, Chennai-600086, India

AnnMarie Hipsley PT PFS PhD
Director of Research Global Vision Research Group Ltd.
ACE Vision Group, PO Box 328
Blacklick Oh, 43004-0328, USA

Ashok Garg MS PhD FRSM
Medical Director
Garg Eye Institute and Research Centre, 235-Model Town
Dabra Chowk, Hisar-125005, India

Athiya Agarwal MD DO FRSH
Consultant
Dr Agarwal's Eye Hospital
19, Cathedral Road, Chennai-600086, India

Barbara Kusa MD
Centre Microchirurgia Ambulatoriale
Via Donizetti, 24, 20052 - Monza, Italy

Carmen Martin-Marcos MD PhD
Ophthalmologic Research Institute
Ramon Castroviejo, Zarracin 25-urb. La. Berzosa
28240-Hoyo de Manzanares, Madrid, Spain

Chaitra Jayadev DOMS
Adityajyot Eye Hospital Pvt Ltd, Wadala
Mumbai-400031, India

David Meyer MB ChB MFGP BSc MMed (Oph) FC Oph PhD
Professor and Head
Deptt. of Ophthalmology, Faculty of Health Sciences
University of Stellenbosch (South Africa)

Dimitrii Dementiev MD
Chief and Medical Director, Blue Eye Centro di, Michro
Chirurgia Oculare Eye Clinic, Arese 20020 (MI)
Via Campo Gallo 21/10, Italy

Fabrizio I Camesasca MD
Deptt of Ophthalmology
Istituto Clinico Humanitas, Rozzano, Milano, Italy

Francesco Carones MD
Medical Director
Carones Ophthalmology Centre, Via Pietro Mascagni, 20
Milan-20122, Italy

Francisco J Gutierrez-Carmona MD PhD
Associate Professor
Ophthalmologic Research Institute
Ramon Castroviejo, Zarracin 25-urb. La Berzosa, 28240-
Hoyo de Manzanares, Madrid, Spain

Franco Bartoli MD
Centro Microchirurgia Oculare
Via Donizetti 24, 20052, Monza, Italy

Frederic Hehn MD
Centre de La Vision, Nations - Vision
23, Boulevard de l'europe, 54500 Vandoeuvre, France

Gene W Zdenek MD
Bellaire Eye and Laser Center, Texas, USA

Georges Baikoff MD
Clinique Monticelli
88, Rue du Commandant Rolland
13008, Marsielle, France

Guillermo Avalos Urzua MD
Terranova NO 676-101, Col. Providencia
Guadalajara, Jal, Mexico, CP 44630

Hijab Mehta MS DOMS FCPS
Adityajyot Eye Hospital Pvt Ltd, Wadala
Mumbai-400031, India

Hitendra Mehta MS
Adityajyot Eye Hospital Pvt Ltd, Wadala
Mumbai-400031, India

JT Lin PhD
4532, Old Carriage Trail, Oviedo, Florida-32765, USA

Matteo Piovella MD
Centro Microchirurgia Oculare
Via Donizetti 24, 20052, Monza, Italy

Roberto Pinelli MD
Director
Istituto Laser Microchirurgia Oculare
Crystal Palace, Via Cefalonia, 70, 25124 Brescia, Italy

S Natarajan MS
Chairman and Medical Director
Adityajyot Eye Hospital Pvt. Ltd.
Plot No. 153, Road No. 9, Major Parmeshwaran Road
Opp. SIWS College, Gate No. 3
Wadala, Mumbai-400031, India

Sunita Agarwal MS DO PSVH
Dr Agarwal's Eye Hospital
19, Cathedral Road, Chennai-600086, India
15, Eagle Street, Langford Town, Bangalore, India

Sylwia McKenzie
Deptt. of Ophthalmology
Faculty of Health Sciences, University of Stellenbosch
(South Africa)

Vivek Kadambi MD DOMS MS
Director
Kadambi Laser Vision Clinic and Research Foundation
Pvt Ltd, 157, Defence Colony
4th Main Road Indiranagar, Bangalore-560038, India

Warren D Cross MD
Bellaire Eye and Laser Center
Texas, USA

Foreword

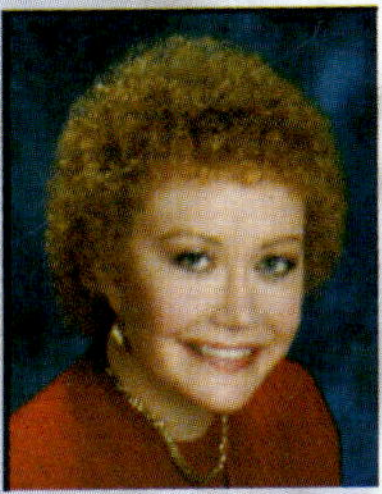

Of all visual defects, presbyopia has been most challenging to correct. Partly because the mechanisms of accommodation and the causes of presbyopia are complex. Presbyopia is also unique in that it is only refractive error that is potentially progressive in nature. The correction of presbyopia remains the holy grail of refractive surgery.

As we all know—many of us to our great chagrin—everyone becomes presbyopic with age. Myopes and higher hyperopes who have always worn glasses may adjust well to bifocal or progressive lenses, contact lens monovision, or other non-surgical solutions. Some people simply don't mind taking reading glasses on and off or carrying around multiple pairs of spectacles. But there is a huge population of individuals who are quite distraught by presbyopia as a very tangible reminder of aging. More than 40% of Americans over age 40, for example, are emmetropes or very low hyperopes who have never worn glasses. Many of these individuals, particularly in the baby boomer generation, are actively looking for a surgical fix to give them back the vision they used to have.

Presbyopia presents challenges for the ophthalmic community. The mechanisms and causes of presbyopia are not fully understood. In fact, competing theories about what is happening to the lens and zonules during accommodation have led to very different supposed cures.

In this *Step by Step Innovations in Presbyopia Management* book, leading experts from around the world discuss presbyopia as a condition and look at appropriate preoperative evaluation of and considerations in recommending innovative treatments for the presbyopic patient.

In this book, authors explore the rich variety of techniques for correcting presbyopia. These include lenticular, corneal, and scleral approaches to restoring accommodation or pseudo-accommodation. Some of them, including conductive keratoplasty and multifocal LASIK, are in widespread use already. Others are still early in the developmental stages. Although I think it is too soon to tell which approach will ultimately find the greatest success, one can find excellent ideas and pearls from the top authorities on the subject in these pages.

While the idea of restoring true, dynamic accommodation is enticing, it is also probably still a long way from fruition. Many will continue to pursue that challenge; but in the meantime, we have some safe and very effective options on the table for restoring to patients what they liked about accommodation—good functional near vision without glasses, and the ability to easily transition from near to distance vision.

I hope you enjoy and learn from this *Step by Step* handy book, and offer my **congratulations to Dr Garg and his fellow editors** for their sincere efforts in compiling such a thorough look at presbyopic surgery.

Dr Marguerite B McDonald
MD
Clinical Professor of Ophthalmology
Tulane University School of Medicine, USA
Medical Director
Southern Vision Institute
New Orleans, Louisiana, USA.
Tel. : (504) 896-1240
E-mail: margueritemcdmd@aol.com

Preface

Presbyopia Management is the ultimate goal for ophthalmologists worldwide. In the 21st century, the innovations and latest developments are taking place in the field of presbyopia. The objective of new innovative techniques is to allow the patient to focus on near objects while retaining his ability to focus on far objects taking into account the refractive errors of the eye when the treatment is performed.

The restoration of reading vision in presbyopia is one of the most important components of modern refractive surgery. For the last five years, a massive innovative work is being done on lenticular, corneal and scleral modifications to correct presbyopia with encouraging results. Multifocal presbyopic LASIK, conductive keratoplasty and multifocal presbyopic lenses are in widespread use already. A lot of work is being done on laser and injectable intraocular lenses for restoration of accomodation with initial success. Use of accommodating implants, multifocal implants, Refractive lens exchange and blended vision implants are lens-based refractive surgery procedures which are quite successful in restoring reading vision in presbyopic patients.

This *Step by Step Innovations in Presbyopia Management* book has been written through a collective effort of leading international presbyopic refractive surgeons with the purpose of providing latest knowledge on modern lens and corneal-based refractive techniques for presbyopia correction to ophthalomologists who are interested in presbyopia surgery practice. Seventeen chapters of this book are written by well-known international refractive surgeons sharing their knowledge and skill covering all aspects of presbyopia management. An interactive CD Rom is being provided with this book showing various operative techniques in presbyopia by master of this field.

We are specially thankful to Shri Jitendar P Vij (Chairman and Managing Director), Mr Tarun Duneja (General Manager, Publishing) and all staff members of M/s Jaypee Brothers Medical Publishers Pvt. Ltd. who extended full cooperation and prepared this high quality international handy book in short time. We are quite hopeful to provide a comprehensive and latest information on presbyopia correction to every interested ophthalmologist and it shall be a useful reference.

Editors

Contents

CD Contents

CHAPTER 1

The Physiology of Presbyopia and its Clinical Relevance

Sylwia McKenzie, David Meyer (South Africa)

DEFINITION

Presbyopia (derived from the Greek word for 'old eye') is a gradual age-related loss in accommodative ability of the eye.

Accommodation is a diopter change in power of the eye to allow near objects to be focused on the retina.

RATE OF LOSS OF ACCOMMODATION

Accommodative loss begins early in life. Objective measurements show 2,3 diopter loss per decade, resulting in a complete loss of accommodation by 50.8 years (Fig. 1.1).[1]

Most of the accommodative amplitude is lost between the ages of 15 and 45.[2]

CHANGES WITH AGE

Ciliary Muscle

- The diameter of the human ciliary muscle decreases with age.
- More connective tissue is deposited. This deposition is probably as a result of rather than a cause of presbyopia. This is borne out by the fact that significant amounts of connective tissue do not occur in subjects still capable of accommodation and accommodative amplitude begins to decline in childhood, long before muscle atrophy would be expected.[7]

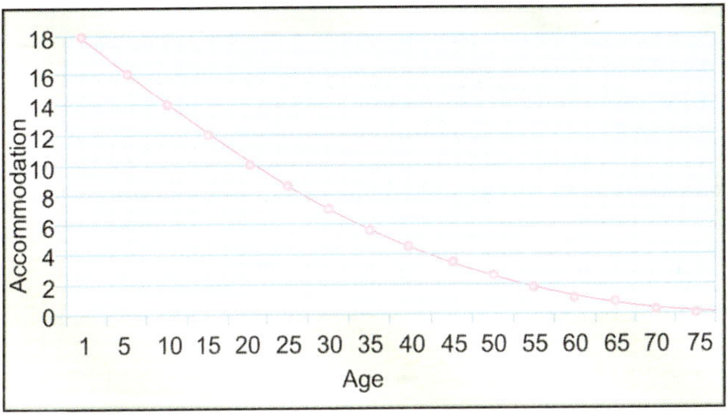

Fig. 1.1: Age-related loss of accommodation[3]

- Recent *in vivo* MRI studies show that:
  1. The *diameter* of ciliary processes does not decrease with increasing age.[7]
  2. No age-dependent change in ciliary muscle *contraction* occurs. The ciliary muscle becomes less responsive due to loss of elasticity of the posterior attachment of the ciliary muscle.[7]
  3. Human ciliary muscle maintains its *mobility* throughout life.[7]
  4. The ciliary muscle apex moves inward and anteriorly with age but no measurable antero-posterior change in ciliary muscle *position* occurs with physiological accommodation.[7]

Choroid

The human choroid retains its elasticity as it is able to bring the cilliary muscle and iris back to their more youthful locations when the age-enlarged lens is removed. This is confirmed by MRI visualization of changing ciliary muscle diameter (ciliary muscle contraction) indicating that a functional choroid must exist to act as the restoring force.[7]

The Lens

Lifelong growth is a defining feature of the crystalline lens, which is formed embryonically from an inverted epidermal layer that constantly generates new cells. The new cells are added onto the surface of the lens and arise from epithelial cells located on the anterior lens surface. The cells elongate, lose all organelles and metabolic apparatus associated with cell growth and division and are displaced inward with new fiber cells growing over them.[7]

Thickness

Both *in vivo* Scheimpflug and MRI imaging show that human lens thickness increases throughout life.[4]

The crystalline lens increases in sagittal thickness right up to adulthood.

The rate of cortical fiber addition slows down to reach the adult rate by about 20 years. At the same time, the central region of the lens stops thickening. Beyond this point in time, increase in the size of the adult lens is due entirely to addition of cortical fiber cells, resulting in linear increase in overall thickness with increasing age.[5]

The Equator Diameter

MRI, which allows for the visualization of the lens equator, enables us to measure the total lens cross-sectional area as well as that of the anterior and posterior portions, by using the equator as the dividing line.

In vivo MRI studies show:

- Both lens thickness and lens cross-sectional area increase with age throughout adult life. This increase is due almost entirely to an increase in the anterior portion of the lens.[7]
- The length of the unaccommodated lens equator is constant with age and has a mean value of approximately 9 mm.[7]
- The accommodated lens equator is smaller than the unaccommodated lens equator, and this difference decreases with advancing age. However, while the accommodated lens equatorial length increases with age, it never exceeds that of the unaccommodated lens equator.

On the basis of these findings, it has been proposed that the reduction of circumlental space seen with advancing age, does not result from an increase in lens equator diameter but rather from the ciliary muscle moving closer to the lens with advancing age.[7]

Shape

Both *in vivo* Scheimpflug and MRI imaging reveal that:

- The anterior curvature of the human lens is less than the posterior curvature.
- The anterior curvature increases with age, while the posterior curvature remains relatively constant.[4]
- Thus, with advancing age, the anterior surface curvature of the human lens approaches that of the posterior. This is consistent with the finding that lens growth primarily affects the anterior portion of the human lens.[7]

Internal Lens Structure

A major advantage of Scheimpflug imaging is the ability to observe changes in regions within the lens nucleus. The following observations have been made:

- The lens nucleus changes with accommodation in the same way as the lens overall; the nucleus is flattest when the eye is focused on infinity and "rounds up" during accommodation. The change in lens thickness along the visual axis during accommodation is due entirely to the change in shape of the lens nucleus, with axial cortical thickness remaining unchanged.[7]
- When the human lens "rounds up", the distance from the cornea to the posterior lens surface is maintained and it is the center of mass that is displaced anteriorly.

The human lens exhibits a continuous gradient of refractive index (GRIN). The refractive index distribution in the human lens is believed to contribute significantly to the total lens power giving the lens an equivalent refractive index which is higher than that of either the nucleus or the cortex and which typically falls in the range between 1.41 and 1.44 depending on age.[6]

Empirical measurements of refractive index distribution done with MRI *(in vitro)* show that refractive index distribution changes significantly with age, with the main change being a decrease in nuclear refractive index. One possibility is that this may occur due to a decrease in soluble lens crystallins in the nucleus. Although no age-related decrease in total lens crystallins has been observed, an increase in water insoluble crystallins with age has been reported, which, is particularly significant in explaining the "lens paradox" (the unaccommodated lens increases in curvature with age; therefore, provided other optical parameters of the eye are constant, the eye would be expected to increase in power, resulting in a myopic shift in refractive error. However, the refractive error of the eye shifts in the hypermetropic direction).[7]

It is interesting to note that even though the age-related changes in the unaccommodated lens shape with age are almost entirely compensated for by an age-related reduction in GRIN, the two processes are, however, not exactly balanced, and overall lens power tends to decrease by 1 diopter with aging.[7]

Lens Biomechanics

It has been proposed that lens "sclerosis" causes presbyopia. This calls into play the definition of sclerosis. If sclerosis is taken to mean *decreased water content,* then recent evidence using Raman micro spectroscopy, *in vitro* MRI and a freeze drying method indicates that:

- Nuclear water content increases with age.
- Water content is not evenly distributed across the lens.
- The behavior of water in the lens is determined in a large part by pressure (both intraocular and accommodative).

In vitro MRI studies of the isolated lens indicate that increasing pressure causes a conversion of free to bound water.[7]

If sclerosis is taken to mean *changes in the mechanical properties of the lens,* then *in vitro* experiments cannot be said to support this theory as accommodative loss begins in childhood and significant mechanical changes in the lens are not seen until after the age at which accommodation is entirely lost.

Lens compression found with *in vivo* MRI is limited to the smaller anterior portion of the lens. The smaller surface area and the thicker anterior lens capsule result in greater compressive forces being applied to the anterior lens material with resting accommodation.

In vitro MRI images of the human lens indicate that the fetal nucleus is primarily located in the posterior portion of the lens. As the fetal and embryonic nuclei are harder than the surrounding adult nucleus, the posterior portion of the lens might remain unresponsive to any pressure from the lens capsule.

Anterior compression decreases with age. This is possibly due to age-related changes in the anterior lens material or due to age-related decrease in zonular tension as the ciliary muscle moves closer to the lens with advancing age.[7]

Lens Capsule

The capsular thickness increases with age. The elasticity of the lens capsule increases until the age of 35 years and then remains constant.[8] These findings dispute the claims that age-related changes in capsular elasticity are sufficient to account for the onset of presbyopia. The force transmitted per unit thickness of the capsule is halved by the age of 60, but the increase in capsule thickness offers some compensation for the loss of elasticity.[2]

Zonules

Scanning electron microscopic studies of human eyes show that with increasing age:

- An anterior zonular/capsular shift on the lens occurs.
- The distance from the zonular/capsule insertion to the lens equator increases.
- The distance from the zonular/capsule insertion to the ciliary processes remains unchanged.

On the basis of the constancy in distance between the zonular/capsule insertion and the ciliary body, it is suggested that there would be no change in zonular length or zonular tension with increasing age, provided the zonular elasticity remained unchanged.

The anterior zonular shift might occur because the posterior capsule is thinner than the anterior capsule and stretches more as the lens continues to grow equatorially within the capsule.

The anterior zonular/capsule shift could also reasonably occur through capsular stretching through an increase in lens thickness.[2]

As a consequence of this zonular/capsule shift, the attachment of the anterior zonular fibers to the lens is anterior to the equator in older eyes. This would result in diminution of the outward directed force on the lens equator by the anterior zonular fibers and is suggested as a contributing factor in presbyopia.[2]

IN VIVO VISUALIZATION OF ACCOMMODATIVE STRUCTURES

Much of the controversy and confusion regarding the mechanism of accommodation and presbyopia has resulted from the difficulty in visualizing the accommodative structures *in vivo* in the intact human eye. The iris prevents visualization of the ciliary muscle and the lens periphery by screening this region from optical methods of visualization. These methods are further complicated by the refractive power of the cornea, which distorts imaging of the remainder of the lens. Invasive methods disrupt the accommodative unit and pharmacological intervention used to increase exposure of the accommodative mechanism affects the iris and ciliary muscle.[7]

The availability of noninvasive imaging techniques has contributed a great deal to uncovering the mechanisms involved in accommodation and presbyopia.

Noninvasive methods available to date:

1. *Scheimpflug slit-lamp photography*
   - Needs to be used in conjunction with appropriate optical correction algorithms
   - Offers high spatial resolution images
   - Can differentiate the lens capsule from the lens material
   - Yields detailed information on lens internal anatomy and its response to both age and accommodation.
2. *High resolution MRI technique*
   - Free of optical distortions
   - Limited in both spatial and temporal resolution, but offers unsurpassed soft tissue contrast (exceeding spatial resolution of traditional MRI).
   - Visualization of entire undistorted human lens and its relationship to the iris, ciliary body and ciliary muscle in any desired imaging plane is possible, without the need to disturb the uveal tract.[7]
3. *Optical coherence tomography (OCT)*

   Provides a two-dimensional graphic representation of light reflected and backscattered from ocular tissue structures, which allows for thickness measurements without contact.[9]

4. *Retro-illumination infrared video photography* and OCT have been used to observe portions of the anterior segment during accommodation, however, both these imaging techniques require the absence of an iris as pigment epithelium blocks the light source's wavelength.

MEASURING OF ACCOMMODATION

Subjective

1. *The "push-up" method*—A near reading chart is moved towards the distance corrected subject until blur is first detected. The reciprocal of the measured distance from the eye to the near reading chart is suggested to represent accommodative amplitude.

   This method generally overestimates true accommodative amplitude. It relies on subjective endpoint criteria (blur), and the patient's interpretation of the task. It is also confounded by the depth of field effects (range of object distances over which there is no detectable change in visual acuity) which are accentuated by accommodative pupil constriction. As target distance decreases, the angle subtended by a given letter size increases, which leads to an overestimation of true accommodative ability. This method can overestimate the accommodative amplitude in a patient with low visual acuity and poor blur detection.[10]

2. *Subjective minus to blur method*—The subject views an illuminated distant letter chart through a phoropter with distance correction in place. Minus lens power is added in 0.25 D steps. The subject reports when the 20/20 line can no longer be held in clear focus. The minus lens power added over the distance correction is recorded as the accommodative amplitude.

   Problems with this method include difference in blur interpretation or task interpretation by subject from one occasion to the next.[10]
3. *Subjective Focometer-induced Accommodation*—A focometer is a monocular Badal optometer similar to a handheld telescope. A manual focusing ring allows the spherical optical power to be increased or decreased; but unlike the stepwise change in power and magnification induced with trial lenses, the Badal principle allows a smooth transition in power with the angle subtended remaining nearly constant. A linear scale on the focusing ring allows the spherical power to be recorded in 0.25 D steps from –8 to +10 D. As minus power is increased, the subject tends to accommodate to overcome the induced defocus. Maximum plus defocus is first introduced into the focometer and the subject instructed to slowly reduce the defocus by adjusting the power with the focus ring until the 20/20 line on a distance reading chart is clearly seen. This spherical power of the focometer is recorded as the

distance refraction. The subject is then instructed to continue adding minus power until the 20/20 line is no longer in focus. This spherical power is recorded and the difference in powers between the two readings is taken as the accommodative amplitude.[10]

Objective

Hartinger Coincidence Refractometer

This optometer measures through a fixed entrance pupil aperture as small as 1 to 2 mm in diameter. The examiner uses a subjective Vernier alignment task to align light mires to measure refraction that is objective with respect to the patient and accurate within 0.25 D. Accommodation needs to be stimulated either with minus trial lenses as subject views a distance letter chart or with Pilocarpine hydrochloride.

Although the Hartinger is no longer generally available, it is commonly used in accommodation experiments. Other refractometers are available, but objective infrared and wave front systems are not generally capable of measuring through the small pupil diameters that result from Pilocarpine stimulation and would not allow the full pilocarpine-stimulated response to be measured.[10]

Pilocarpine

Pilocarpine (2% or 6%) is a parasympathomimetic agent that causes both iris and ciliary muscles to contract which leads to meiosis and accommodative spasm. When accommodation is pharmacologically stimulated, an involuntary accommodative response takes place that is not accompanied by convergence eye movements (usually coupled with voluntary accommodation). Even if a little accommodation is present, it can be stimulated with Pilocarpine.

When accommodation is pharmacologically stimulated and measured with an objective instrument, minimal cooperation and no voluntary accommodative effort is required from the subject. This method may be very important for testing the results of accommodative restorative procedures if preoperative and postoperative test results are compared with normal controls.[10]

In phakic subjects physiological accommodation does not cause anterior ciliary muscle displacement, whereas pharmacologically induced accommodation in pseudophakic subjects causes anterior displacement of both the iris root and ciliary muscle.[7] Thus, pharmacologically induced accommodation may overestimate the amount of pseudoaccommodation that occurs with physiological accommodative effort (Fig. 1.2).

The dynamic components of accommodation include:

a. *Latency* (time between the target onset and response onset).
b. *Time constant* (time taken for the response to attain 63% of the new steady-state amplitude).

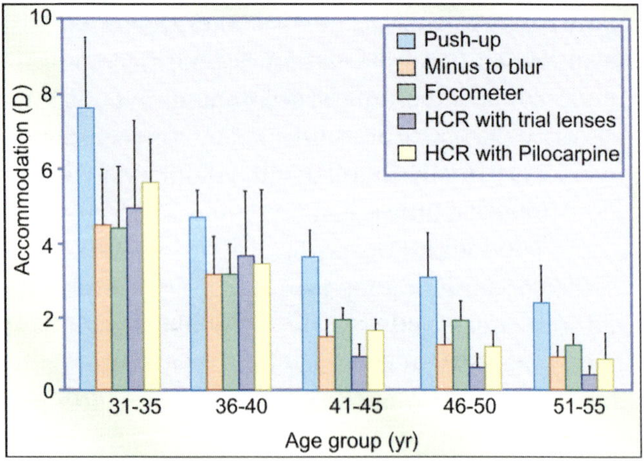

Fig. 1.2: Mean maximum accommodative amplitudes for the various methods of accommodation measurement[10]

c. *Main sequence* (relationship between response amplitude and its correlated peak velocity)
d. *Accommodative oscillations:* These measurements can be helpful as they describe the sequence of events leading up to a focused image. Upon sensing and processing a defocused retinal image, a neuromotor command is generated and transmitted to the ciliary body. This initiates the appropriate deformation of the crystalline lens and change in refractive power resulting in an improvement of the overall optical quality and clarity of the retinal image.[11]

   In presbyopia:

   - Latency for accommodation increases as a function of age. This increased processing time for the accommodative response is speculated to result from delay in central higher-order neural processing time, rather than peripheral neuromuscular transmission delays.

- The time constant for accommodation is independent of age, thus the lens changes in shape at the same speed in old and young subjects.
- The main sequence does not change with age suggesting lack of any gross neurological system deficit, and furthermore confirming relatively normal lens biomechanics.
- With advancing age, mean amplitude of oscillation becomes attenuated, (both high and low frequencies decreased) reflecting changes in the lens (and capsule) viscoelastic properties.[11]

THEORIES OF PRESBYOPIA

Lenticular (Helmholtz) Theory (Fig. 1.3)

- The crystalline lens becomes harder with age.
- The lens substance can no longer be moulded into an accommodated state by the lens capsule when the resting zonular tension is released.
- The hardened lens substance is incapable of being pulled into a flattened and unaccommodated state by the zonular tension and is in a fixed state and unable to undergo accommodative change.

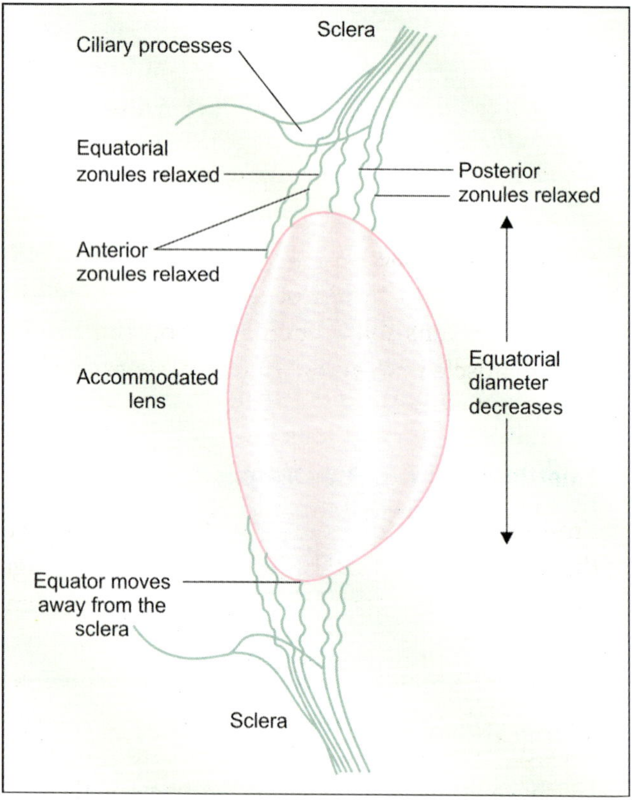

Fig. 1.3: Helmholtz theory of accommodation. The ciliary muscle contracts, all the zonules relax, the lens rounds up as a result of its elasticity, and the equatorial diameter of the lens decreases[12]

Problems with this theory:

1. If the zonules simply relax , the entire lens equator would be expected to drop posteriorly when supine

and the lens would be unstable during near vision which has not been shown to happen.

2. An increase in spherical aberration is also expected since a more uniformly spherical lens creates a greater separation between the peripheral and central point of focus. On the contrary, this has been shown to decrease.
3. A myopic shift should occur as the progressive increase in lens mass encroaches on the zonule-ciliary muscle with aging. In fact, a hyperopic shift occurs with age.[3]

Geometric Theory of Presbyopia

- Presbyopia is a consequence of altered geometry of the lens/zonular relationship with increasing age, due to the anterior zonular shift when the crystalline lens thickens.
- As anterior zonular shift occurs, the angle between the anterior zonules and the lens anterior surface is altered. As a result, the zonular fibers transmit a nearly tangential force to the surface of the lens when the ciliary muscle contracts and the zonules relax, so the relaxation of the zonules has very little effect on the capsule and hence the shape of the lens.
- This theory tries to explain presbyopia in the absence of changes to lens elasticity or ciliary muscle degeneration.[2]

Problems with this theory:

The presbyopic lens is suggested to be in an unaccommodated form. How the altered geometry prohibits the lens from accommodating but can provide the necessary force to keep the lens in an unaccommodated form is not explained.[2]

Schachar's Theory of Presbyopia

- Schachar's theory of accommodation is utilized.
- It suggests that continued lens equatorial growth is the cause of presbyopia.
- The age-related growth of the lens equator decreases the distance between the lens and ciliary body, thus slackening zonular tension such that accommodative effort fails to increase the zonular tension sufficiently to actively pull on the lens equator (Fig. 1.4).

Problems with this theory:

1. The lens diameter measured *in vivo* in human eyes has been shown to be age independent.
2. The resulting zonular tension would cause more accommodative microfluctuations in older eyes as a result of reduced stability of the lens. However, the accommodative microfluctuations are more pronounced in young eyes and almost absent in people with presbyopia.[2]

Disaccommodation Theory of Presbyopia

- Presbyopia is not caused by a failure of the lens to accommodate, but rather by a gradual failure of the lens to be held in an unaccommodated form at rest.[2]

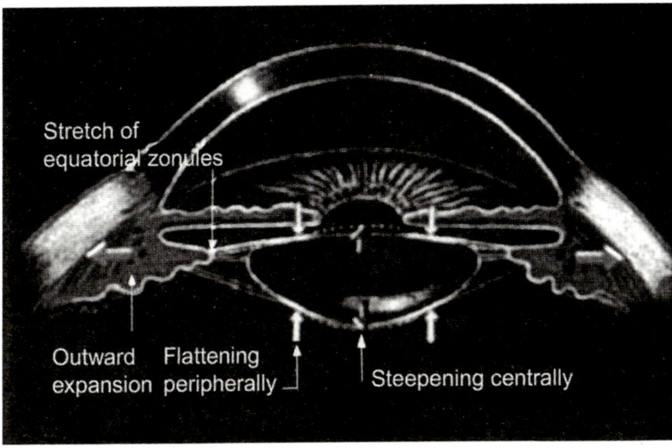

Fig. 1.4: Equatorial zonular stretching causes central steepening and peripheral flattening of crystalline lens illustrating Schachar's theory[3]

- The failure is due to:
  1. an increased growth and altered diameter of the lens.
  2. altered zonular/lens geometric relationships.
  3. age changes in ciliary muscle position.
  4. loss of elasticity of the choroid which prevents the application of the correct zonular tension to hold the lens in its unaccommodated state.[13]
- The lens progressively assumes a more accommodated configuration until eventually it is in a fully accommodated state and no further accommodation can take place.

Problems with this theory:

1. Neither increasing nor decreasing the zonular tension can alter the elderly crystalline lens focal length.

2. The shape of the nucleus of the presbyopic lens is unlike that of the young accommodated lens.

Multifactorial Theory of Presbyopia

Proposes that the accelerated loss of accommodation relative to other physiological indicators of age, is due to the combined effect of normal age-related changes in the component elements of the accommodative apparatus.[14]

Problems with this theory:
The assumptions used in the model proposed were based on data that has no empirical backing and could be manipulated to draw different conclusions than those presented in the model.[15]

Modified Geometric Theory

- The most recent model proposed by Strenk et al (2004).
- Describes the effect of lens growth on accommodative loss as follows:
  1. The pupillary margin of the iris rests on the anterior surface of the lens and upward forces applied by the lens to the iris are translated to the iris root and ciliary muscle.
  2. Scleral curvature produces a tangential force, causing an inward as well as anterior displacement of ciliary muscle and the iris root, thus reducing the pupil diameter.

3. This brings the pupillary margin closer to the thickest part of the anterior lens surface, thus amplifying the effect of lens thickness on iris root and ciliary muscle anterior/inward displacement and the cycle continues as the lens grows.
4. As the ciliary muscle moves upward and inward with age, circumlental space is reduced, resulting in decreased zonular tension.
5. A reduction in zonular tension during resting accommodation leads to both increased lens curvature and reduction in lens accommodative response.
6. This theory also provides a possible mechanism for the development of senile meiosis.
7. This theory is based on information from *in vivo* MRI studies and is consistent with the following observed age-related changes:
   - reduction of circumlental space
   - anterior/inward displacement of the ciliary muscle
   - anterior/inward displacement of the iris
   - lack of lens equatorial growth
   - significant increase in lens thickness
   - cross-sectional area and curvature
   - decrease in lens compression
   - undiminished ciliary muscle contraction.[7]

Problems with this theory:

1. As discussed with the Helmholtz/lenticular theory, it does not explain how the lens remains stable

during near vision if the zonules supporting it are relaxed during accommodation.

2. A myopic shift would be expected.
3. Objections to proposed relaxation of zonules with ciliary muscle contraction during accommodation.

CURRENT TREATMENT MODALITIES FOR PRESBYOPIA

The principal aim of treatment is not necessarily to restore accommodation but to allow those individuals who have lost accommodation physiologically to cope without glasses.[16] The current treatment options include optical correction with spectacles or contact lenses. Monovision whereby one eye is corrected for distance and the other for near can be achieved by contact lenses, refractive surgery or intraocular lenses.

Surgical options include multifocal intraocular lenses either in the anterior or posterior in the chamber. Scleral expansion band surgery, however, has thus far generated controversial results.

The methods of presbyopia correction to date have only offered a partial approximation of the focusing ability of the younger eye. These are "static" corrections and compromise on many aspects of vision such as limited diopter range of clear vision, reduced image contrast and impaired stereoscopic vision. The real goal is to restore to the patient the "dynamic eye" of controllable continuously adjustable power, ideally covering at least a three dioptric range between normal reading and distance infinity.[17]

REFERENCES

1. Koretz JF et al. Accommodation and presbyopia in the human eye: aging of the anterior segment. Vision Res 1989;29:1685.
2. Kaufman PL, Alm A. Adler's Physiology of the eye, 10th edn. 2003;214.
3. Harmer RH. The Surgical Reversal of Presbyopia: a new procedure to restore accommodation. Ophthalmic Practice 2000;18(5):210-14.
4. Koretz JF et al. Scheimpflug and high-resolution magnetic imaging of the anterior segment: a comparative study. J Opt Soc Am A Opt Image Sci Vis 2004;21(3):346-54.
5. Koretz JF et al. The zones of discontinuity in the human lens: development and distribution with age. Vision Res 1994;34(22):2955-62.
6. Moffat BA et al. Age-related changes in refractive index distribution and power of the human lens as measured by magnetic resonance imaging *in vitro.* Vis Res 2002; 42:1683-93.
7. Strenk SA et al. The mechanism of presbyopia. Progress in Retinal and Eye Research 2005;24:379-93.
8. Krag S, Andreassen TT. Mechanical properties of the human lens capsule. Prog Retin Eye Res 2003;22(6):749-67.
9. Wirbelauer C et al. Imaging scleral expansion bands for presbyopia with optical coherence tomography. J Cataract Refractive Surg 2003;29:2435-38.
10. Ostrin LA et al. Accommodation measurement in a prepresbyopic and presbyopic population. J Cataract and Refractive Surg 2004;30:1435-44.
11. Mordi JA et al. Dynamic aspects of accommodation: age and presbyopia. Vis Res 2004;44:591-601.

12. Scachar RA. The correction of presbyopia. International Ophth Clinics 2001;41(2):53-70.
13. Tamm E et al. Age-related loss of ciliary muscle mobility in the rhesus: role of the choroid. Archives Ophth 1992; 110:871.
14. Weale RA. Why we need reading-glasses before a zimmer frame. Vis Res 2002;40:2233-40.
15. Glasser A. Letter to the Editor; Vis Res 2001;41:3083-87.
16. Baikoff G. Surgical treatment of presbyopia: scleral, corneal, and lenticular. Curr Opin Ophthalmology 2004; 15:365-69.
17. Charman WN. Restoring accommodation to the presbyopic eye: how do we measure success? J Cataract Refract Surg 2003;29:2251-54.

CHAPTER 2

Patient Selection and Preoperative Examination in Presbyopic LASIK—An Important Step

Francisco J Gutiérrez-Carmona,
Carmen Martín-Marcos (Spain)

INTRODUCTION

Now-a-days, refractive surgery is largely optional for myopia, hypermetropia and astigmatism. The majority of patients decide to take the option of surgery encouraged by the positive results experienced by a familiar or friend.

This surgery requires from the refractive surgeon the establishment of a selective indication for each patient, which will mean that occasionally the surgeon will have to exclude a patient interested in surgery.

During the first appointment with the patient, an ophthalmological medical examination should be carried out. This will determine the refractive technique indicated in each case and the problems contra-indicating surgery. In this appointment, we should ask the patient what has motivated him to take the option of surgery, and inform him about the refractive procedure to be carried out. Finally, we should decide which option to proceed with.

Normally, the patient is informed as to the method of refractive surgery, it is important for the expected postoperative results and for informed consent.

MEDICAL HISTORY

The majority of refractive errors found in patients can be corrected by glasses or contact lenses, solutions involving no risk to the patient.

During the first appointment, the patient's filiation data must be noted, such as: name, occupation, age, address, general condition and state of ophthalmological refraction.

Motivation

The main objective which motivates a patient to undergo refractive surgery is to achieve partial or total independence from his refractive disorder. The commonest reasons given in an interview with a patient are:

- Independence from use of glasses. The use of glasses in some occupations is limiting.
- Intolerance to the wearing of contact lenses. The patient may have difficulty in the daily manipulation of contact lenses, problems with hypersensitive reaction to contact lens cleaning solutions, or with dry eye, giant papillar conjunctivitis or keratitis.
- Professional reasons. Access to certain professions is determined by a required level of uncorrected visual acuity (army, fire-brigade, police, pilots, etc.).
- Aesthetic reasons.
- Sport-related reasons.

On the other hand, another motive for carrying out LASIK would be to improve visual results after performing previous ocular surgery.

For example, after radial keratotomy, cataract surgery or penetrating keratoplasty.

A careful selection of the patient must be taken into consideration, and an explanation of the risks and benefits of LASIK.

Age

In general, the patient should have a minimum age of 21 years for LASIK, as this assures a certain refractive stability. However, the professional motivation of some patients may require the age limit to be lowered.

Refraction

Prior to surgery, the patient should have had refractive stability for at least a year and a half to two years. If a patient has had refractive changes in recent years, surgery is not indicated.

The wearing of hard or gas-permeable contact lenses should be discontinued two weeks before refraction. Soft contact lenses can be worn until 3 days before surgery.

Ocular Pathology

Inflammatory and infectious diseases of the cornea, such as ophthalmic herpes zoster and herpetic keratitis.

Previous cataract or retinal ocular surgery does not contraindicate surgery, but it may cause peroperative complications.

Previous cornea transplant surgery increases the risk of complications, including rejection.

Refractive surgery by radial keratotomy will depend on the state of the cornea and on the number of incisions. Lamellar refractive surgery does not contraindicate LASIK.

Systemic Pathology

The patient should be asked if he is diabetic, as such patients may present changes or oscilations in refraction or evidence of incipient cataracts. Surgery is not indicated for these patients.

Collagen diseases are contraindicated; although in some inactive cases, LASIK can be carried out.

Surgery is not indicated in the case of psychic disorders or mental deficiency.

Some drugs used to treat diseases produce alterations in the tear film. For example, in young patients the most frequent is atopia and the use of antihistamines. Also, the use of anticholinergics in the treatment of depression. These situations are relative contraindications.

LASIK

Indications

Specific Indications

- We recommend keratomileusis *in situ* with excimer laser for young patients with stable accommodation and myopia no greater than –10.00 diopters.

For patients with myopias more than –10.00 diopters, phakic lenses are indicated.

For patients close to presbyopic age with high myopia, we should consider transparent lens surgery with the implantation of a low-power posterior chamber IOL.

- Low and moderate hypermetropias from +1 to +5 diopters.
- Astigmatism up to 5 diopters.
- Corneal casts with stable topography and refraction.
- Keloids.
- Difficulty in the postoperative follow-up of the patient.
- Patients contraindicated by the use of corticosteroids.
- Frustrated keratoconus. In patients with normal pachymetry, similar topographical maps in both eyes and aged over 35.
- Diabetes.

Relative Indications: Surgical Difficulties

- Small corneal diameter.
- Keratometry of less than 41 diopters.
- Corneal epithelial fragility.
- Narrow parpebral fissure.
- Small and deep orbit.
- Corneal neovascularization. Common in myopes with contact lenses.
- Previous surgery of the:
  — Retina: detachment, vitrectomy.

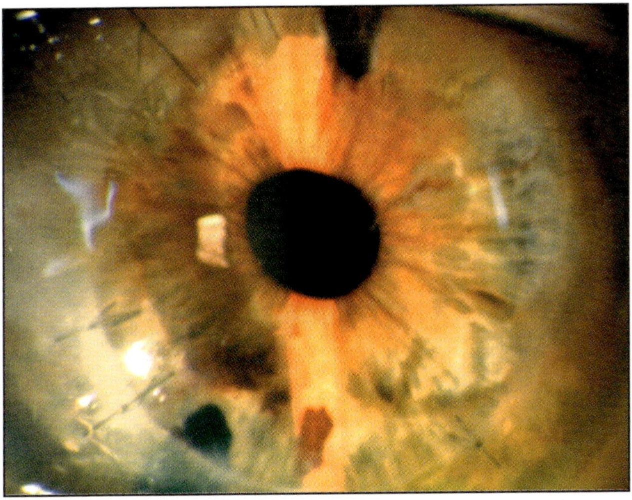

Fig. 2.1: Penetrating keratoplasty

— Cornea: keratoplasty (Fig. 2.1), radial keratotomy.
— Lens: cataract.

- Conjunctival alterations. Pterygium.

Contraindications

- Single eye.
- Corneal dystrophies. Endothelial alterations, cornea guttata, dystrophies and ruptures of Descemet's membrane (Fig. 2.2).
- Herpes simplex.
- Collagen diseases.
- Keratoconus (Figs 2.3 and 2.4).
- Reduced pachymetry.

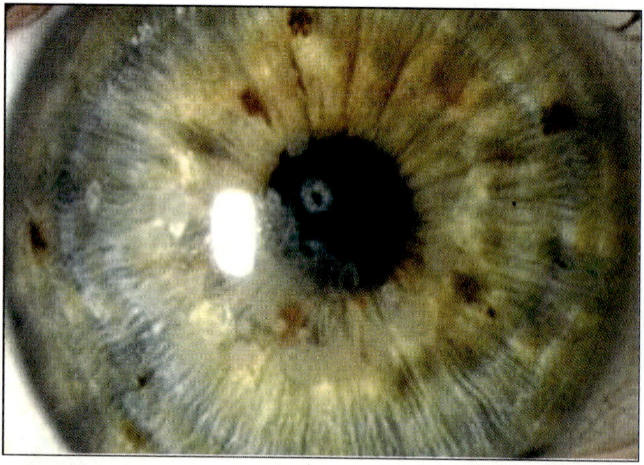

Fig. 2.2: Granular corneal dystrophy

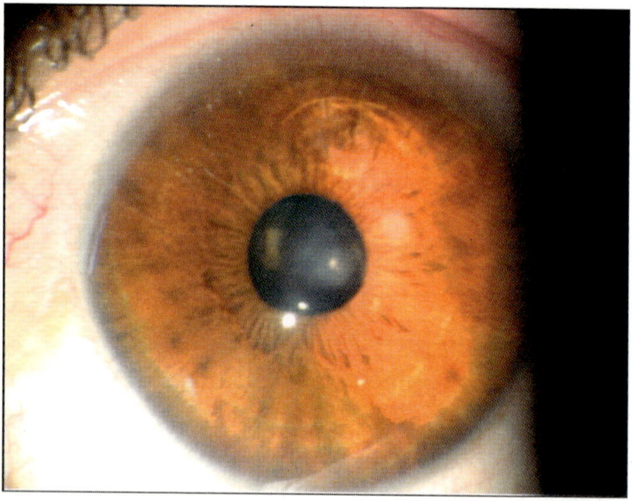

Fig. 2.3: Keratoconus

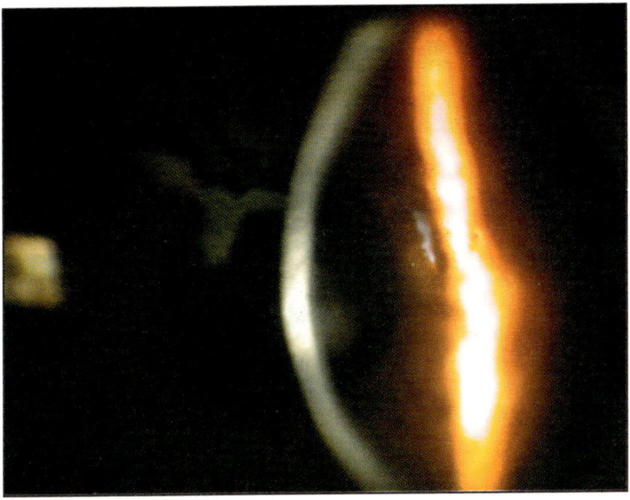

Fig. 2.4: Keratoconus

Preoperative Examination

Patient selection for LASIK often determines the overall success of the procedure; therefore, it is crucial that a thorough preoperative examination be performed, accompanied by appropriate counseling.

Contact lens wear should be discontinued prior to the examination; 3 days for soft contact lens wear and 2 weeks for rigid gas permeable lenses.

A complete eye examination, including manifest and cycloplegic refraction, slit-lamp examination, dilated fundus examination, and corneal topography (Fig. 2.5), is recommended. In addition, an estimate of scotopic pupil size is helpful in screening candidates that may be at risk for postoperative glare.

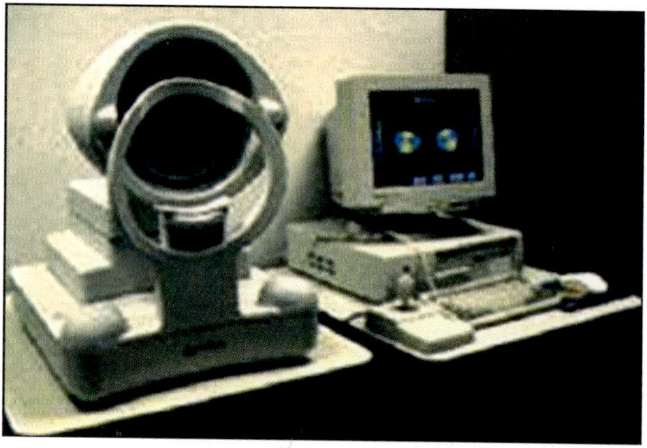

Fig. 2.5: Corneal topographer

Poor surgical candidates include patients with a refraction out of the recommended correction range, patients with active inflammation of the external eye or iritis, and patients with cataracts or retinal holes or tears. Although LASIK surgery has only rarely been associated with vitreoretinal pathology, retinal detachments following surgery have been reported. Therefore, screening with indirect ophthalmoscopy is advisable.

The refraction should be stable prior to performing surgery. Stability can be assessed by serial refractions and an evaluation of medical records and old glasses. Any change more than 0.50 diopters compared to the above is suspect and suggests that the current refraction is not stable.

Corneal topography is essential to rule out keratoconus and irregular astigmatism. These problems tend to make the surgical outcome unpredictable. In particular, keratoconus patients may be more prone to the development of ectasia or thinning following LASIK; refractive surgery on this group of patients is considered investigational. Corneal topography also is helpful in evaluating contact lens-induced corneal warping. Patients with irregular corneas and a history of contact lens wear should be observed with serial refractions and topography until both stabilize.

Finally, ultrasonic pachymetry is necessary to determine if enough corneal thickness is present to create a flap, ablate the cornea, and still leave enough tissue behind to prevent structural weakening and ectasia. Current guidelines recommend leaving at least 250 μm of cornea untouched.

REFERENCES

1. Gimbel HV, Penno EE. Patient Selection and Preoperative Workshop. In Gimbel HV, Penno EE (Eds): LASIK Complications: Prevention and Management. Thorofare, NJ: Slack Inc 1999:11-19.
2. Gutiérrez-Carmona FJ, Martín-Marcos C. Patient selection for photorefractive keratectomy (PRK) and laser *in situ* keratomileusis (LASIK). In Agarwal S, Agarwal A, Pallikaris IG, Neuhann TH, Knorz MC, Agarwal A (Eds): Refractive Surgery. New Delhi: Jaypee Brothers Medical Publishers (P) Ltd. 2000;40-43.

CHAPTER 3

Pre-LASIK Retinal Examination and its Clinical Relevance

S Natarajan, Chaitra Jayadev,
Hijab Mehta, Hitendra Mehta (India)

INTRODUCTION

The Eye Disease Case-Control Study Group in its study on the "risk factors for idiopathic rhegmatogenous retinal detachment"[1] has determined that an eye with a spherical equivalent refractive error of –1 to –3 diopters has a fourfold increased risk of retinal detachment compared with a non-myopic eye. If the refractive error was more than –3 diopters, the risk is increased 10-fold. The data suggest that almost 55 percent of non-traumatic detachments in eyes without previous surgery are attributable to myopia. LASIK has proven to be an effective procedure for correcting these very same low-to-high myopes. There are relatively few reports on vitreoretinal complications in comparison with anterior segment complications associated with LASIK.[2,3] Considering the large number of LASIK being done today, even these cases can amount to a significant visual insult. Keeping that in view it, an evaluation of the posterior segment of the eye (vitreous and retina) via binocular indirect ophthalmoscope is a must to rule out possible retinal diseases prior to scheduling a LASIK.

METHODS OF RETINAL EVALUATION

Indirect ophthalmoscopy with 360 degrees scleral depression and/or 3 mirror contact lens examination. While performing scleral indentation, maximum

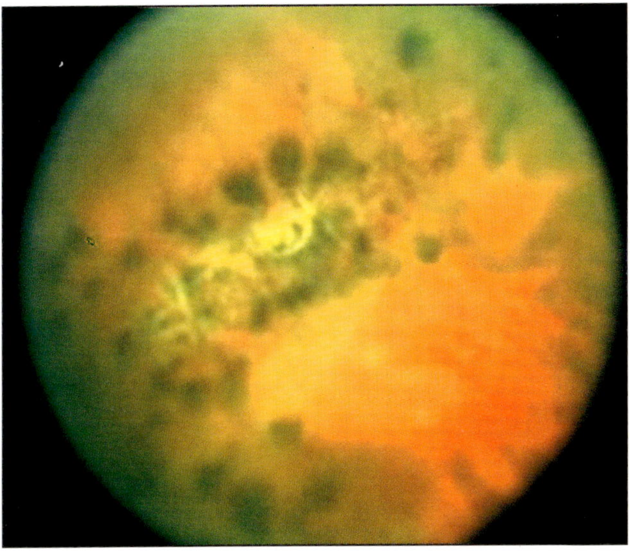

Fig. 3.1: Lattice lesion containing small atrophic holes

dilation is of utmost importance, this will greatly improve the ability to see the indented retina. As a rule, scleral indentation is performed through the lids. However, there are times when one will have to use an anesthetic and place the depressor directly on the sclera to get a better view. A 3 mirror contact lens examination with a slit-lamp may accomplish adequate examination without scleral depression and serve to stabilize the eye in an uncooperative patient. Whatever the method used, the clinician has to make sure that the entire 360 degrees of the retinal periphery is well evaluated for any treatable lesions.

WHAT IS THE RISK?

It has been known for long that myopia is associated with an increased incidence of retinal detachments.[1] Lifetime risks were 0.2 percent in hyperopes, emmetropes, and myopes with refractive errors of as great as –1.00 D, but the risk increased to 7 percent for eyes with more than –9.00 D of refractive error.[6] The incidence of these risks in eyes undergoing LASIK has been studied with one study[4] illustrating a 0.02 percent yearly incidence in patients who had an average

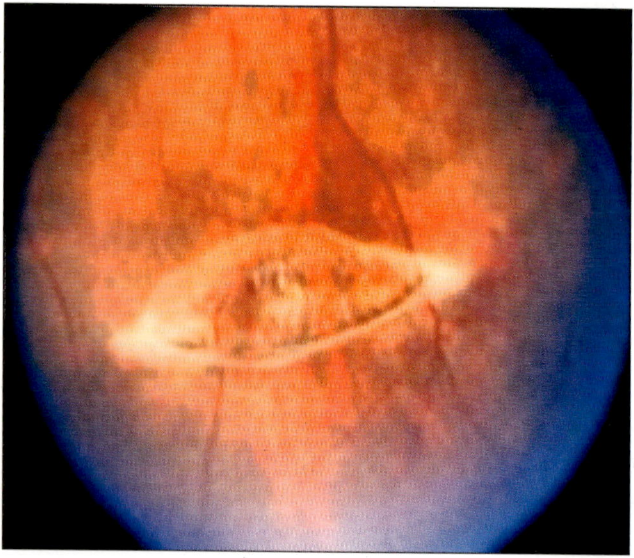

Fig. 3.2: A peripheral lattice lesion demonstrating the typical snail-track appearance, with overlying vitreal opacities (which may represent glial proliferations or regions of increased vitreoretinal condensation)

refractive error of –6.00 D, a finding that indicates a lack of association between LASIK and retinal detachment, while few other studies indicate a higher association. However, no large, long-term, case-controlled, prospective study has yet been undertaken to produce convincing associations.

MECHANISM OF RETINAL CHANGES DURING LASIK

Ozdamar in 1998 and Tsai in 2001[7,8] published the case reports of two patients with RD due to giant tears, who have had their onset respectively 2 and 9 months after LASIK refractive correction. These patients had medium-to-high myopia. These authors ascribed an important role to the mechanic stress on the vitreous base caused by the microkeratome during the aspiration phase. In fact, during this surgical phase, the ocular tone increases over 65 mm Hg. The fast change in the ocular tone during the aspiration alters the shape with a remarkable increase of the equatorial diameter and traction on the vitreous base with the eventual development of peripheral tears. This pathogenetic mechanism is very similar to that of contusive trauma. Other mechanisms of trauma during LASIK may include excimer laser-induced shock waves (pressure as high as 100 atm) caused by the high number of energy pulses required to achieve adequate surgical results in moderate and high myopes.[4,5]

Another study found that one (2%) of 50 patients with refractive errors of less than –4.00 D and five (10%)

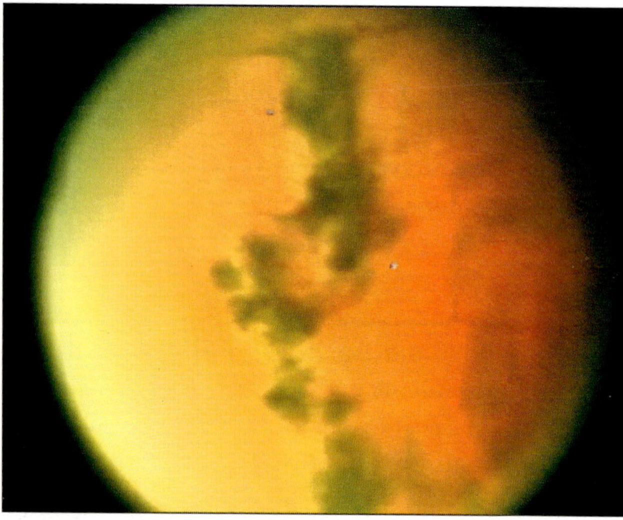

Fig. 3.3: An example of a heavily pigmented lattice lesion

of 50 patients with refractive errors of more than –7.00 D developed a PVD shortly after undergoing LASIK.[9] It has also been suggested that a delayed posterior vitreous detachment (PVD) from premature vitreous liquefaction associated with myopia can account for the time delay between the LASIK procedure and the development of an RRD.[5] In another study, 78 percent of the retinal breaks occurred in the temporal quadrant, a finding that could be attributed to the additional pressure that the microkeratome applied on the temporal side of the eyes.[4]

On the other hand, many ophthalmologists believe that the retinal detachments observed after LASIK are not related. They opine that these detachments are more due to the effects of myopia than LASIK. The time delay between the LASIK procedure and incidence of RRD goes against any direct causation, although a delayed PVD may be a contributing factor. Supporting this school of thought is a study, which has found that, for all cases in which retinal tears led to a detachment, the retinal detachment occurred within 6 weeks of the development of the retinal tears unlike in the case of post-LASIK detachments (average of 5 to14 months).[10]

Keeping in mind the large PVD frequency in high myopes of younger ages and the association of PVD with an increased risk of RRD, any PVD and subsequent RRD in a post-LASIK patient could simply be due to a spontaneous PVD that is unrelated to the prior LASIK surgery.

In addition, ocular pneumoplethysmography—the study of more than 69,000 tests of ocular blood flow using a device that applies suction to the globe to create IOPs in excess of 100 mm Hg—has never been shown to create a retinal detachment. Additional biomechanical studies on pneumoplethysmography patients have illustrated minimal eye wall displacement and vitreous disturbance.[12]

IS PROPHYLACTIC PHOTOCOAGULATION A MUST?

Many ophthalmologists recommend prophylactic photocoagulation and routinely make their LASIK patients undergo a thorough retinal examination prior to the LASIK procedure.[4] Supporting this protocol is the study with the lowest incidence of RRD, in which every patient underwent a thorough retinal evaluation and prophylactic photocoagulation treatment if needed, prior to the LASIK procedure.[4]

Albeit this, there have been no prospective studies directly comparing prophylactic treatment versus no treatment or those showing any definite reduction in the incidence of rhegmatogenous detachments in patient's asymptomatic retinal lesions. On the other hand, there have been clinicians who have documented that the risk of retinal detachment in eyes with significant myopia or lattice degeneration is not altered by prophylactic treatment; and, therefore, the procedure is not indicated because its long-term complications are unknown.[13,14]

Although it is assumed that LASIK induces some form of trauma and thereby causes detachments, it is known that eyes with lattice degeneration are not at an increased risk of detachment after a traumatic injury.[6]

Even if a patient has a treatable lesion and does undergo photocoagulation for the same, it does not ensure that the risk of retinal detachment is mitigated. In the eventuality of a post-LASIK detachment, the surgeon is left with a dilemma of whether or not to use a scleral buckle to treat the condition. On the one hand, it is the most appropriate form of treatment and on the other, it nullifies the effect of the LASIK procedure by inducing a myopic shift.

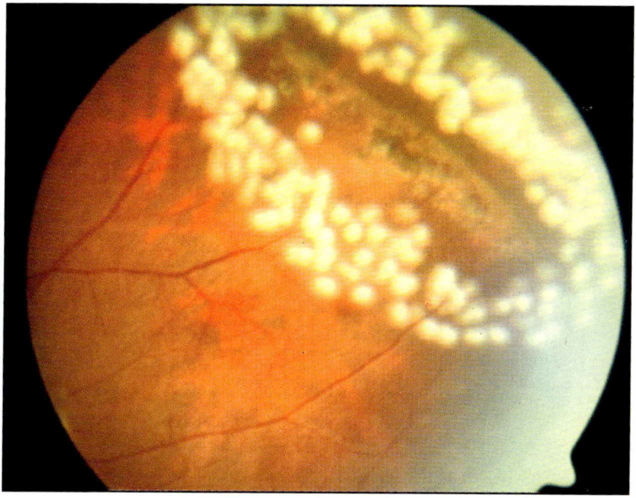

Fig. 3.4: Lasered lattice

A patient requiring laser photocoagulation for a treatable retinal lesion, should be scheduled for LASIK at least 2 weeks after the laser treatment.

CONCLUSION

Until large-scale prospective studies are undertaken to prove that an association exists between LASIK and retinal detachments, the use of prophylactic photocoagulation will remain physician-dependent. In the present scenario, it seems most prudent to have patients undergo a dilated fundus examination prior to LASIK; symptomatic breaks and all horseshoe tears should receive treatment, but the value of treating asymptomatic operculated or atrophic holes is unknown.[11] Finally, even if a patient undergoes refractive correction using LASIK, the eye is inherently myopic and, therefore, requires annual retinal check and reporting to a retinal surgeon on an emergency basis if symptoms occur.

REFERENCES

1. The Eye Disease Case-Control Study Group. Risk factors for idiopathic rhegmatogenous retinal detachment. Am J Epidemiol 1993;137:749-57.
2. Chan CK, Arevalo JF, Akbatur HH, et al. Characteristics of 60 myopic eyes with pre-laser *in situ* keratomileusis retinal examination and post-laser *in situ* keratomileusis retinal lesions. Retina 2004;24:706-13.
3. Arevalo JF, Ramirez E, Suarez E, et al. Incidence of vitreoretinal pathologic conditions within 24 months after laser *in situ* keratomileusis. Ophthalmology 2000;107: 258-62.
4. Arevalo JF, Ramirez E, Suarez E, et al. Rhegmatogenous retinal detachment in myopic eyes after laser *in situ* keratomileusis: frequency, characteristics, and mechanism. J Cataract Refract Surg 2001;27:674-80.
5. Aras C, Ozdamar A, Karacorlu M, et al. Retinal detachment following laser *in situ* keratomileusis. Ophthalmic Surg Lasers 2000;31:121-25.
6. Burton TC. The influence of refractive errors and lattice degeneration on the incidence of retinal detachment. Trans Am Ophthalmol Soc 1989;87:143-55.
7. Ozdamar A, Aras C, Sener B, Oncel M, Karacorlu M. Bilateral retinal detachment associated with giant retinal tear after laser-assisted *in situ* keratomileusis. Retina 1998;18(2):176-77
8. Tsai YY, Lin JM, Tsai SC. Giant tear retinal detachment after laser *in situ* keratomileusis—a case report. Kaohsiung J Med Sci 2001;17(11):586-89.

9. Luna JD, Artal MN, Reviglio VE. Vitreoretinal alterations following laser *in situ* keratomileusis: clinical and experimental studies. Graefe's Arch Clin Exp Ophthalmol 2001;239:416-23.
10. Davis MD. The natural history of retinal breaks without detachment. Trans Am Ophthalmol Soc 1973;71:343-72.
11. Comer G, Ciulla T. Is there a connection between LASIK and RRD? Cataract Refract Surg Today 2003;29-31.
12. Mazur Do, Hollifield R, Gee W. Retinal detachment in myopic eyes after laser *in situ* keratomileusis (comment). Am J Ophthalmol 2000;129:824-25.
13. Byer NE. Long-term natural history of lattice degeneration of the retina. Ophthalmology 1989;96:1396-1401.
14. Wilkinson CP. Evidence-based analysis of prophylactic treatment of asymptomatic retinal breaks and lattice degeneration. Ophthalmology 2000;107:12-15.

CHAPTER 4

Humanoptics Accommodating IOL for Presbyopia Correction

Sunita Agarwal, Athiya Agarwal,
Amar Agarwal, Ashok Garg (India)

INTRODUCTION

There are basically three methods to correct presbyopia.[1] The first comprises surgeries done on the sclera. This includes techniques like scleral bands or anterior ciliary sclerostomy. The second comprises surgeries done on the cornea like presbyopic LASIK or conductive keratoplasty. The third and most widely performed are surgeries done on the lens. This includes multifocal IOLs and the accommodating IOLs.

HUMANOPTICS

Humanoptics[2] is a company in Germany, which has developed a pseudophakic accommodating foldable IOL. This is the Humanoptics akkommodative 1 CU IOL, which helps correct both distance and near vision based on Helmholtz's theory. This lens was developed on the work done by Khalil Hanna MD using finite element computer models.

AKKOMMODATIVE 1 CU IOL

This lens, which is an accommodating IOL, is a hydrophilic acrylic lens with a refractive index of 1.46. It has an integrated ultraviolet (UV) inhibitor. The lens has four square edge dynamic transition elements (Fig. 4.1) with an overall diameter of 9.8 mm and a biconvex optic of 5.5 mm. It comes in a diopter range of +16 to +26 D in 0.5 D increments. The lens functions by

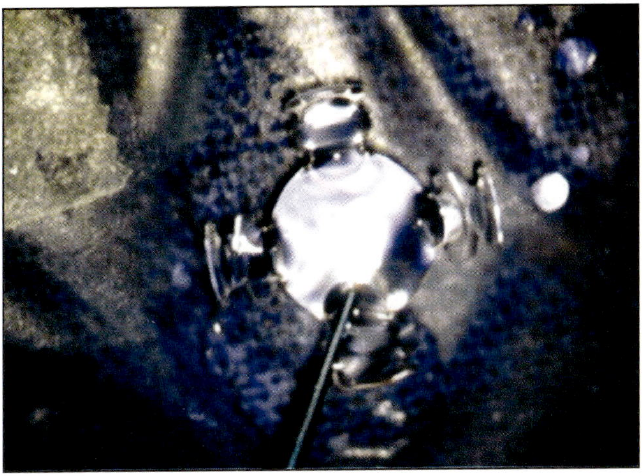

Fig. 4.1: The Humanoptics Akkommodative 1 CU IOL. Note the four haptics present in the lens, which have a hinge connection to the optics

dynamic transition elements that enable the optical power of the lens to change during accommodation.

MECHANISM OF ACTION

With the Akkommodative 1 CU inserted into the bag, stimulus of accommodation leads to contraction of the ciliary muscle and relaxation of the zonules. The resultant mechanical energy stored in the capsular bag is transmitted to the implant during accommodation. This leads to a specific posterior deformation of the implant that increases its optical power, allowing near objects to focus on the retina. When accommodation ends, the ciliary muscle relaxes and zonular tension increases. The capsular bag is stretched and the Akkommodative IOL returns to its unaccommodative state. This results in distant objects being focused on the retina.

BIOMETRY

If one uses an ultrasonic device, the measurement probe is applied directly to the anterior surface of the cornea. Due to the induced contact pressure the value of the axial length measurement may be smaller. It is thus recommended to add an average contact factor of 0.2 mm to the measured axial length. The K-readings are to be used in millimeters and not in diopters as this can create an impact in the calculations. The target refraction should be 0 to –0.5 D.

SURGICAL TECHNIQUE

The Humanoptics lens comes in a sterile package and is an acrylic hydrophilic IOL. The lens is taken from the package using a special forceps (model RS 211 from Humanoptics). This lens is the placed in a special cartridge (model RS 420 from Humanoptics). The lens is placed in such a way that the four haptics of the lens are outside the cartridge flange. Then using the same forceps parallel pressure is applied to fold the lens and the cartridge is partially closed. The forceps is then slowly removed and used to place the haptics into the loading chamber. When correctly positioned and

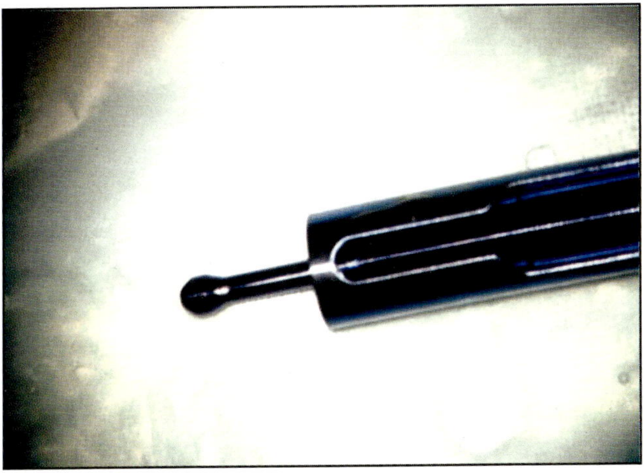

Fig. 4.2: The Humanoptics injector

ascertained that the lens and haptics are completely in the tunnel, the wings can be fully closed. Using the other end of the same forceps, which has a special lens loader, the lens is pushed into the cartridge tunnel. For this, one should apply light and constant pressure until the entire length of the loader is inserted into the cartridge. The cartridge is then placed in the injector (Fig. 4.2) (model RS 310 from Humanoptics).

The cartridge is now pushed in the positioning slot as well as down to ensure that the tunnel runs parallel to the tip of the injector. The lens is now ready (Fig. 4.3) to be implanted simply and reliably by slowly pushing the piston of the injector. The right hand holds the injector and the cartridge is passed through the incision inside the anterior chamber (Fig. 4.4). The

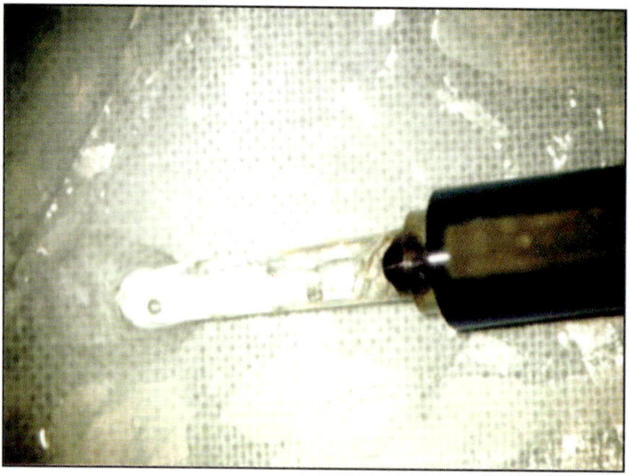

Fig. 4.3: The cartridge is loaded onto the injector

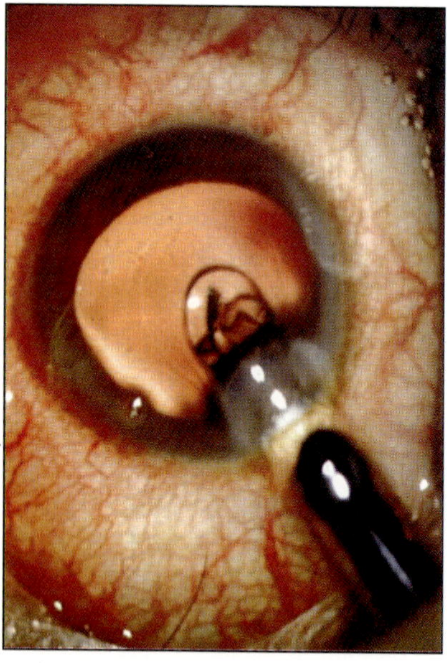

Fig. 4.4: Cartridge inserted inside the eye. The lens is gradually implanted

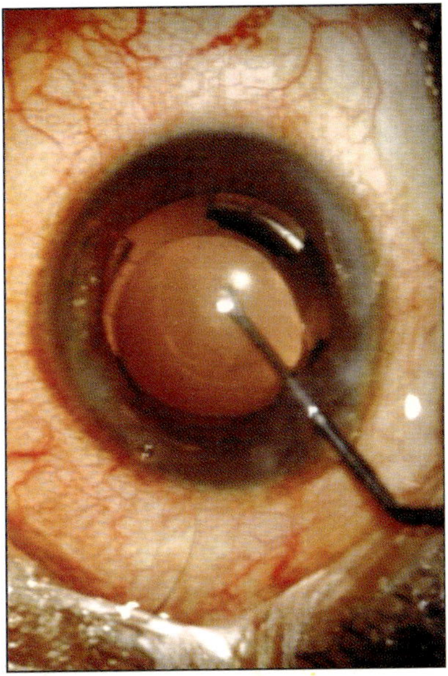

Fig. 4.5: The lens haptics are placed in the capsular bag using the Agarwal globe stabilization rod (Gueder, Germany)

incision size is 3.2 mm. The lens is gradually inserted inside the anterior chamber. The four haptics lie on top of the rhexis. Then using an Agarwal globe stabilization rod from Gueder (Germany), each of the four haptics is placed inside the capsular bag (Fig. 4.5). Once the entire lens is in the capsular bag (Fig. 4.6), the viscoelastic is removed by the irrigation-aspiration probe.

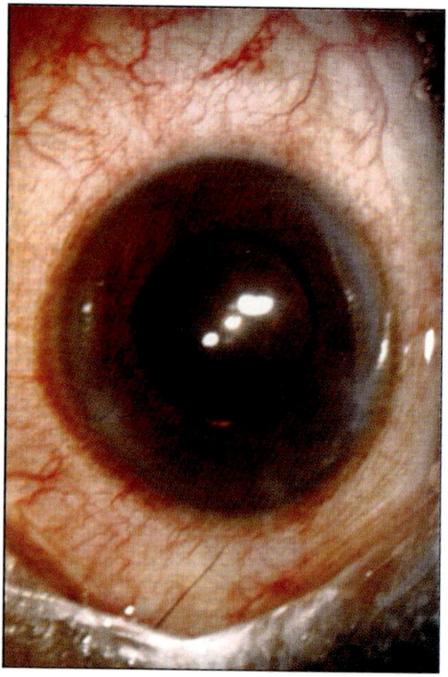

Fig. 4.6: The Accommodating IOL is entirely in the capsular bag

POSTOPERATIVE CARE

The accommodative potential will be achieved after complete capsular bag shrinkage. This takes about a month after surgery.

REFERENCES

1. Agarwal A. Presbyopia: A Surgical Textbook. Slack; 2002, USA.
2. Gregory Pamel J. The Humanoptics Akkommodative 1 CU IOL in A Agarwal's Presbyopia: A Surgical Textbook. Slack; 2002, USA; 211-214.

CHAPTER 5

Pseudoaccommodative ReSTOR IOL to Correct Defocus and Presbyopia in Refractive Lens Exchange

Francesco Carones (Italy)

INTRODUCTION

Refractive lens exchange (RLE) is becoming the predominant procedure to correct ametropia in the presbyopic age, particularly in eyes where the crystalline lens is not totally transparent. Traditional monofocal IOLs have been used at this aim, and refractive results proved satisfactory. However, monofocal IOLs give the patients only one optimal focusing distance, either at distance, intermediate or near, while vision at all other distances has to be optimized with traditional spectacle correction. More recently, the introduction of multifocal and accommodative IOLs gave the patients more focusing options for being less dependent on spectacle correction. Current status of refractive lens exchange has been recently described by Hoffman et al,[1] while potential risk factors, especially in highly myopic eyes, were reported by Ravalico et al.[2] Hoffman et al,[3] Dick et al,[4] and Packer et al[5] discussed the use of multifocal IOLs for refractive surgery purposes, while Montes-Mico et al described changes in contrast sensitivity after multifocal intraocular lenses implantation.[6,7] More recently, Kuchle et al described the refractive results from eyes that received accommodative IOLs.[8]

The introduction of a new multifocal, diffractive/ apodized IOL stimulated my interest in assessing its clinical results when implanted for refractive surgery purposes during RLE. This IOL adds a +3.20 D correction to the nominal dioptric power. At this purpose, a trial was set involving eyes with virtually no lens opacity, from patients asking for refractive surgery. This was a prospective consecutive interventional case series study, including thirty eyes from 15 patients (9 females, 6 males). Age ranged between 45 and 62 years (mean 51.5 years). Uncorrected and best-corrected visual acuity at distance, intermediate and near, refraction, wavefront analysis and psychometric testing were assessed.

All the patients had either mild hyperopia or mild myopia (that was due to the limited IOL dioptric power range available, ranging +18.00 to +25.00 D) and asked for refractive surgery. All of them presented with presbyopic features requiring additional near spectacle correction when using either distance spectacle correction or contact lenses. Exclusion criteria were: unavailability of the IOL dioptric power to bring the eye plano, pre-existing ocular pathology, history of previous refractive surgical procedures, pre-existing astigmatism more than 1.00 D, patient unrealistic expectations. All patients were visited before and after surgery at the Carones Ophthalmology Center, Milan, Italy, where surgery was also performed in an outpatient ambulatory fashion.

All eyes were implanted with the Alcon AcrySof ReSTOR IOL (Figs 5.1 and 5.2). This is a 6.0 hydrophobic acrylic IOL with a central 3.6 mm diffractive pattern surrounded by a monofocal portion, giving the IOL an apodized structure. The diffractive pattern

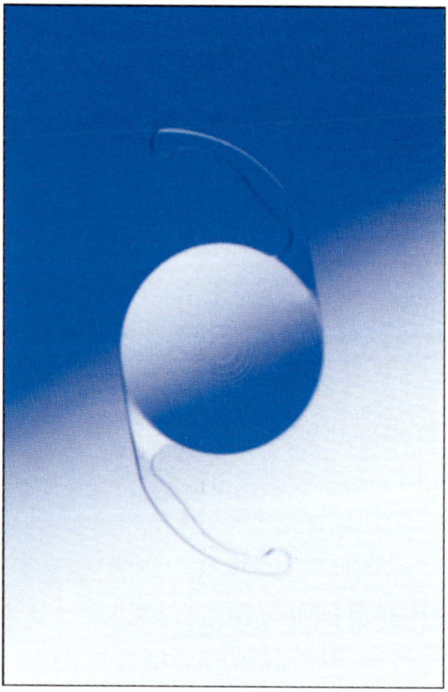

Fig. 5.1: The AcrySof ReSTOR IOL diffractive/apodized pattern

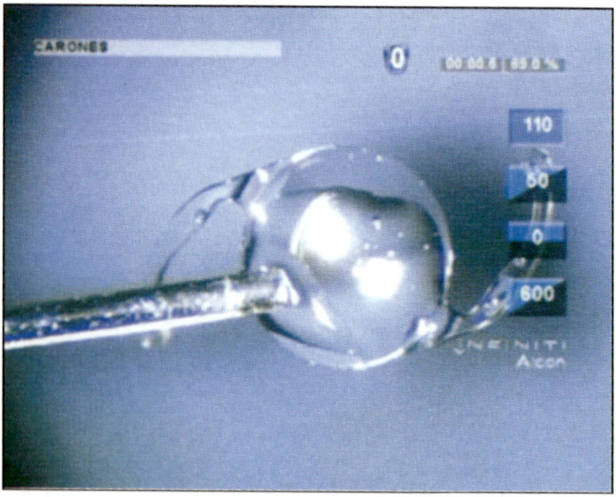

Fig. 5.2: The ReSTOR IOL

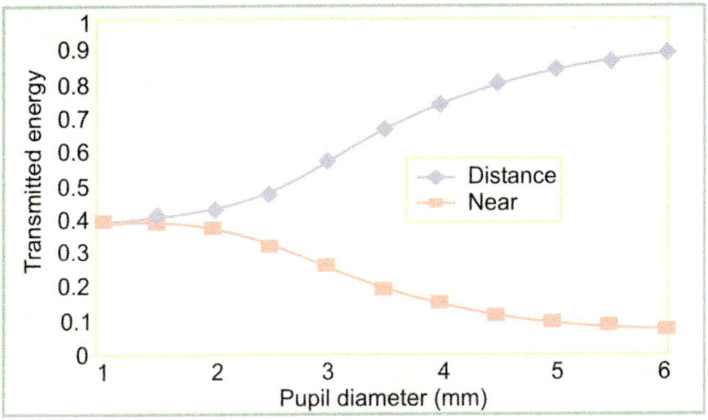

Fig. 5.3: Light transmission through the ReSTOR IOL

provides two main focal points, with a +4.00 D additional power to the nominal one (3.2 D at spectacle plane). The apodization is intended to enhance light transmission at the distance focal point when pupil dilates, as shown by Figure 5.3.

All surgeries were performed under topical anesthesia. The lens material was removed by aspiration only without any ultrasounds, then the IOL was implanted in the capsular bag through a 2.8 mm limbal temporal tunnel using Monarch C cartridge and Asico Royale injector. One single-stitch 10/0 nylon suture was placed for astigmatism control purposes in eyes having more than 0.50 D with-the-rule pre-existing astigmatism. Adverse effects and complications were assumed to be assessed at all postoperative visit and recorded in a specific part of the data collection form. We reported none. Manifest refraction, uncorrected and best spectacle-corrected high-contrast visual acuity were tested by ophthalmologists at 4 m distance using Snellen projected charts, and at 60 and 30 cm using Jaeger charts. Wavefront analysis was performed by optometrists using the Alcon LADARWave aberrometer; and to avoid false readings from the edge of the IOL, analysis was performed over a 6.0 mm pupillary diameter. All these parameters were assessed before surgery and at all postoperative follow-up visits. A questionnaire was used to assess psychometric testing, and this was done before surgery and at one, three and six months. Postoperative examinations were scheduled on day one and three after surgery, and then at two weeks, one, three and six months.

All surgeries were uneventful. All the implanted IOLs were in the capsular bag, with no meaningful decentration relative to the pupillary aperture (Fig. 5.4). Six months after surgery, manifest refractive spheroequivalent error (MRSE) was ± 0.62 D in all eyes. Uncorrected visual acuity was 20/25 or better in all eyes, and no eyes reported with best-corrected visual acuity loss. At 30 cm, all patients could read J2 or better, and all of them but one could read J4 or better at 60 cm. Figure 5.5 presents the binocular intermediate and near vision once distance was corrected.

Wavefront analysis did not disclose any significant increase in high-order aberrations: mean preoperative root mean square (RMS) was 0.32 microns before surgery and 0.34 microns at six months ($p= 0.11$); mean

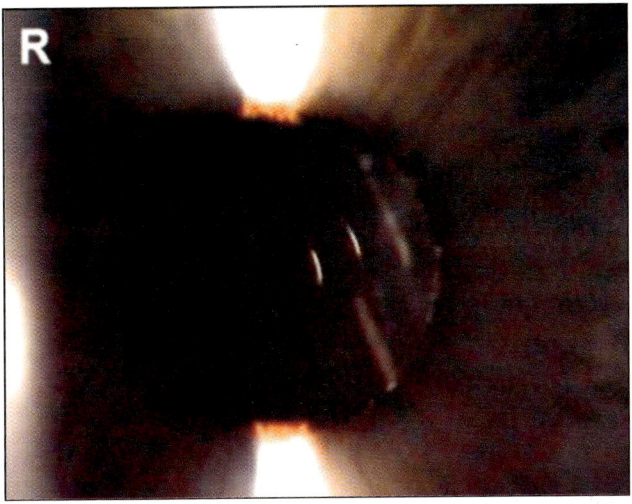

Fig. 5.4: Clinical image of an implanted ReSTOR

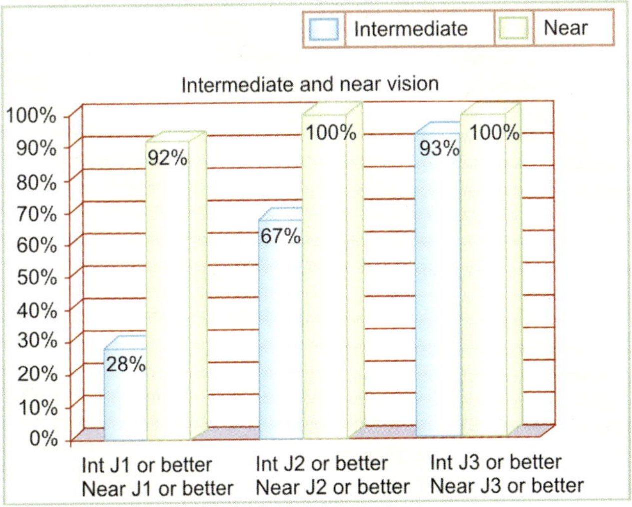

Fig. 5.5: Intermediate and near vision

spherical aberration was 0.18 microns before surgery and 0.16 microns at six months (p= 0.12).

Psychometric testing assessed at six months disclosed all 15 patients as happy and all of them would have the procedure done again. Fourteen patients are not using spectacles at all, while the one using them does it for intermediate, computer-working distance. None of the patients reported any visual complaints at bright illumination, none of them reported severe night-visual symptoms, while two of them described only slight visual symptoms at dim-light illumination (ghost imaging, starbusts). Those visual disturbances were reported more frequently at one (seven patients) and three months (four patients), thus showing a trend to decrease.

These results indicate refractive lens exchange using the ReSTOR IOL as an effective surgical procedure to correct pre-existing low levels of spherical ametropias (due to the current limited range of dioptric power available) and ReSTOR an extremely satisfactory near distance visual acuity in those patients being in the presbyopic age. The ReSTOR has two principal focusing points, of which one is intended to be used for distance (the nominal IOL power), the other is for reading purposes, i.e. 30 to 35 cm from the eye (3.2 D power at spectacle plane). All that is in between these two main focal points receives less light energy, thus representing the theoretically weaker focusing distances; particularly, less light energy is transmitted by the IOL for that distance around 60 cm which is commonly used for working with computers, or for reading the speed-gauge when driving. Both our measurements and patients subjective testing reported this intermediate as less effective than reading- or infinity distance. Although we did not evaluate defocus curve, all the patients could read at least J4 at 60 cm, and only one of them required spectacle correction to increase his visual performance when using computers.

One of the most interesting features of this diffractive IOL consists of the apodization. This means that the IOL transmits more light energy for the distance focal point as the pupil dilates, to improve vision and decrease night-vision symptoms when pupil dilates. Although we did not perform any contrast sensitivity tests or low-contrast visual acuity assessment, wavefront analysis did not disclose any increase in high-order aberrations as measured before and six months after surgery; and the psychometric subjective evaluation we performed was extremely encouraging, with no patients reporting severe side effects or visual symptoms from contrast sensitivity reduction.

The subjective psychometric testing also revealed that the potential night-vision symptoms like haloes, starbusts and ghost images, were only slight and not meaningful when referred; and most important, they decreased during follow-up, meaning that some kind of brain process in excluding the second, out-of-focus image, has an important role for the IOL better performance. However, we believe that an accurate patient selection with the exclusion of those hyper-critical patients having unrealistic expectations and/or too many visual demands (hard computer workers, professional night-drivers, etc.), may help in achieving high satisfaction levels from the patients.

To the best of our knowledge, there is no peer-reviewed literature regarding the results of the ReSTOR IOL implanted during refractive lens exchange, while this IOL is under FDA investigation for implant during cataract surgery. Other studies on multifocal and accommodative IOLs implanted either during cataract surgery or during refractive lens exchange have been published.[3-8] Zonal refractive IOLs like the AMO Array, showed to provide satisfactory results in terms of spectacle independence, but they also disclosed some limitations like the reading performance under bright-light conditions, as well as reduction in contrast sensitivity and induction of visual disturbances (haloes, glare, starbusts, ghost images) under mesopic and scotopic conditions. Our series of patients did not complain of bright-light reading performances, nor about severe night-vision disturbances. Accommodative IOLs provided excellent distance performances, while near vision showed to be not as effective as with our series of eyes implanted with the ReSTOR.

Refractive lens exchange still imply some potential risks. Endophthalmitis is certainly the most important;

and, compared to laser or surface procedures, with intraocular surgery this is certainly amplified. However, small incision lens surgery, wide-spectrum local antibiotics, and adequate pre-postoperative care have minimized the incidence of this complication. Crystalline lens removal has also been associated with a higher risk of retinal detachment. This is particularly true for highly myopic eyes,[2] that were not included in this study, and posterior capsule opacification (PCO) with consequent Nd:YAG laser capsulotomy.[9] Although this series of patients may be at higher risk of PCO due to the relatively young age, we did not see any even early trace of PCO in these eyes over the follow-up that extends over a one year period. Additionally, the hydrophobic acrylic material the IOL is made of,[10] and the barrier effect of the square-edge design, proved to be particularly effective in avoiding PCO. Needless to say, further studies with longer follow-up are necessary to definitely assess the long-term safety of the procedure.

In conclusion, we believe the ReSTOR IOL is an extremely effective device to provide the patients undergoing refractive lens exchange with a full range of uncorrected vision, without the induction of clinically significant side effects or visual symptoms. With accurate patients' screening and selection, this IOL may become the standard of care not only for refractive surgery purposes but also in cataract surgery.

REFERENCES

1. Hoffman RS, Fine IH, Packer M. Refractive lens exchange as a refractive surgery modality. Curr Opin Ophthalmol 2004;15:22-28.
2. Ravalico G, Michieli C, Vattovani O, Tognetto D. Retinal detachment after cataract extraction and refractive lens exchange in highly myopic eyes. J Cataract Refract Surg 2003;29:39-44.
3. Hoffman RS, Fine IH, Packer M. Refractive lens exchange with a multifocal intraocular lens. Curr Opin Ophthalmol 2003;14:24-30.
4. Dick HB, Gross S, Tehrani M, Eisenmann D, Pfeiffer N. Refractive lens exchange with an array multifocal intraocular lens. J Refract Surg 2002;18:509-18.
5. Packer M, Fine H, Hoffman RS. Refractive lens exchange with the array multifocal intraocular lens. J Cataract Refract Surg 2002;28:421-24.
6. Montes-Mico R, Espana E, Bueno I, Charman WN, Menezo JL. Visual performance with multifocal intraocular lenses: mesopic contrast sensitivity under distance and near conditions. Ophthalmology 2004;111:85-96.
7. Montes-Mico R, Alio JL. Distance and near contrast sensitivity function after multifocal intraocular lens implantation. J Cataract Refract Surg 2003;29:703-11.
8. Kuchle M, Seitz B, Langenbucher A, et al. Comparison of 6-month results of implantation of the 1CU accommodative intraocular lens with conventional intraocular lenses. Ophthalmology 2004;111:318-24.
9. Colin J, Robinet A, Cochener B. Retinal detachment after clear lens extraction for high myopia: seven-year follow-up. Ophthalmology 1999;106:2281-84.
10. Vasavada AR, Raj SM. Anterior capsule relationship of the AcrySof intraocular lens optic and posterior capsule opacification: a prospective randomized clinical trial. Ophthalmology 2004;111:886-94.

CHAPTER 6

Multifocal Phakic Implant for the Correction of Presbyopia

Georges Baikoff (France)

INTRODUCTION

Correcting presbyopia is an essential challenge for refractive surgery. This particular type of surgery is not so much to do with restoring accommodation, but more a question of giving patients an opportunity of living without spectacles for distant and near vision. This opens the door to a number of compromises or alternatives to real accommodation surgery.

Presbyopia affects most people over the age of 45 and if we consider that in the United States 50 percent of the population is presbyopic,[1] through extrapolation, this represents several billion individuals throughout the world.

Considering the degree of ametropia (high/low myopia, high/low hyperopia, emmetropia) several options are available. Unilateral myopization (monovision) of the dominant eye or multifocal correction of either the cornea or crystalline lens, either by adding a new lens or exchanging the crystalline lens if it is still transparent.

A choice is, therefore, available to both surgeons and patients as not one of all these techniques provides the perfect solution; and in the years to come, it is quite probable that several different but complementary solutions will be available. We decided to work on three possible options: the cornea, the crystalline lens and the sclera and will give the results we obtained following implantation of a bifocal lens for correcting both slight ametropia and an average presbyopia of + 2.50 D.

NEWLIFE BIFOCAL PHAKIC IMPLANT

The bifocal refractive phakic IOL is an anterior chamber angle-supported lens marketed under the trade name of NEWLIFE (**Ioltech**)* . The optic is of soft 28 percent hydrophilic acrylic, the haptic is of polymethyl-meth-acrylate (PMMA), and the footplates at the extremities are of hydrophilic acrylic. The 5.5 mm diameter optic is divided into 3 zones: the center, which is for distance vision, the medium periphery which is for near vision; and the periphery which is for distance vision. The central zone diameter is 1.50 mm, and the near intermediate zone is 1.1 mm wide (Figs 6.1 and 6.2). The haptic is shaped like the number 2 and is available in overall diameters of 12.0 mm, 12.5 mm and 13.0 mm.

The IOL comes in powers between –5.00 D and + 5.00 D for distant vision with a single addition of +2.50 D for near vision. This addition is a compromise, allowing a slight overcorrection for 50-year-old subjects and a slight undercorrection for 60-year-old subjects; these slight refractive inaccuracies will prove to be generally well accepted.

ANTERIOR CHAMBER DIMENSION

Internal Diameter

For all angle-supported implants, it is essential to carry out a precise evaluation of the internal diameter of the

*__Ioltech__, Avenue Paul Langevin, BP 5 17053 La Rochelle, France, Tel + 33 5 4644 8550 ; Fax + 33 54644 8560

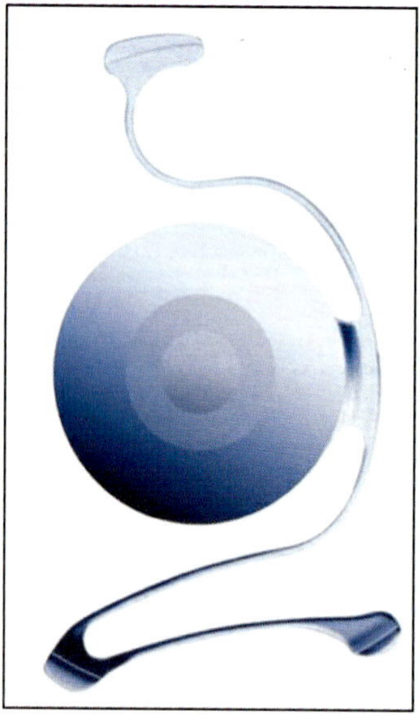

Fig. 6.1: Drawing of presbyopic anterior chamber implant (*Courtesy:* Elsevier)

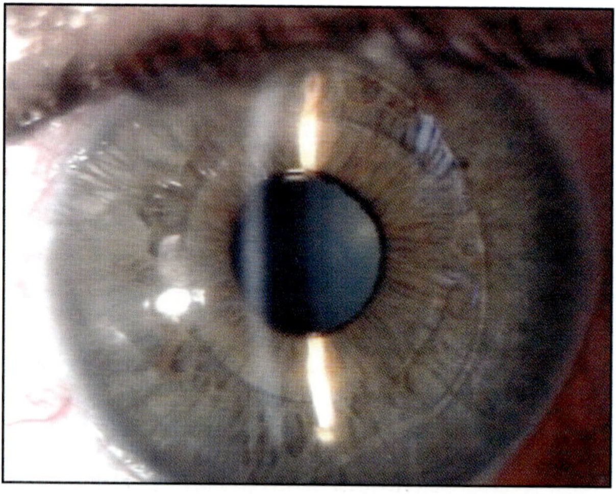

Fig. 6.2: Postoperative aspect (*Courtesy:* Elsevier)

anterior chamber. We began by using the white-to-white method, then we used a PMMA-graduated sizer which was inserted into the anterior chamber during surgery. In fact, all these measurements are relatively approximate; and for an implant to remain stable in the anterior chamber, it must not only be adapted to the eye's largest diameter in order to avoid rotation but also as near as possible in size to this diameter so that there is no pressure on the iris which in the long run gives rise to pupil ovalization.

These problems cannot be solved with the actual ultrasound A and B-scan techniques. However, modern imaging techniques such as the Artemis, ultra-high frequency ultrasound equipment and the anterior segment OCT give more precise measurements of the anterior chamber's internal diameter. We were able to demonstrate *in vivo*, and this was confirmed by Liliana Werner on cadaver eyes, that in 75 percent of cases, the anterior chamber's internal vertical diameter was bigger than the horizontal one. In daily practice, we therefore, systematically preoperatively measure the anterior segment helping us in the choice of implant (Fig. 6.3).

Anterior Chamber Depth

Minimum anterior chamber depth must be equal to or above 3.1 mm (measured from the corneal epithelium to the anterior surface of the crystalline lens). This is of course, a safety notion but does not, in fact, take into account the implant's vault (Fig. 6.4).

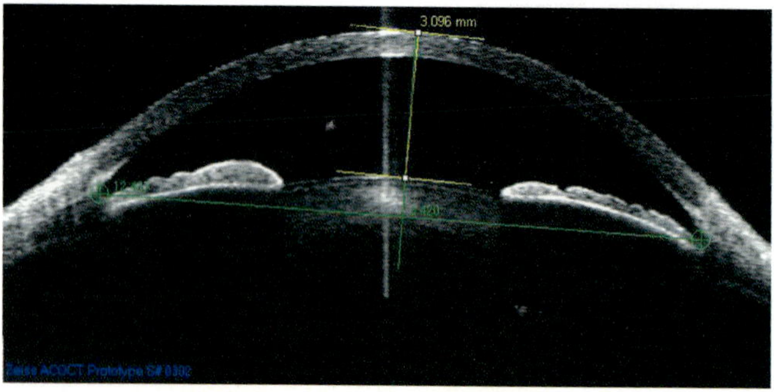

Fig. 6.3: AC measurements with the Visante™ OCT prototype (*Courtesy:* Elsevier)

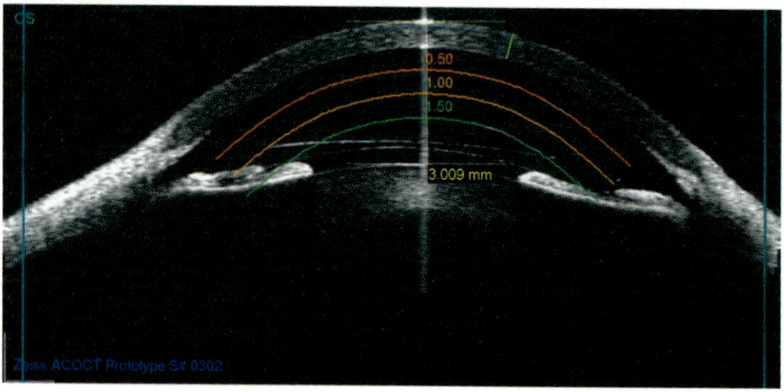

Fig. 6.4: Endothelial safety distances (*Courtesy:* Elsevier)

SURGICAL TECHNIQUES

Topical, local regional or general anesthesia was used based on the surgeon's or patient's choice. Surgery (Fig. 6.5) is relatively simple and consists in placing the lens, which is folded at the time of surgery, into the anterior segment of the eye in front of the iris.

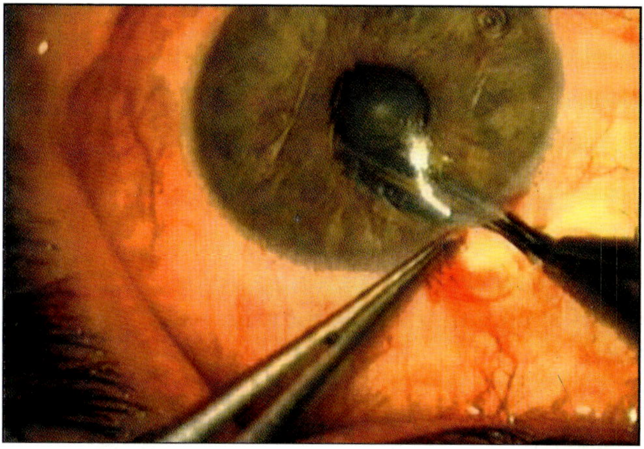

Fig. 6.5: Insertion of the implant with optic folded in three (*Courtesy:* Elsevier)

A preoperative myosis is essential (preoperative installation of 2 percent Pilocarpine drops). A corneal or corneoscleral incision is carried out with a 2.8 mm calibrated knife. Viscous substance was injected into the anterior chamber, two paracenteses were made at 3 and 9 o'clock positions to allow subsequent maneuvers in the anterior chamber.

The lens is folded into three with a special folder before being inserted. First, the two leading footplates are introduced into the anterior chamber followed by the optic and trailing haptic. Once the lens is in the anterior chamber, pressure on the forceps is gently released and the optic unfolds. When the lens is open in the anterior chamber and depending on the largest axis, the implant will be rotated to fit this axis. It is essential that all the viscous substance is removed at the end of surgery to avoid postoperative hypertonia with URRETS ZAVALLA syndrome (fixed dilated pupil). The viscous substance is replaced with BSS. No sutures are required with the self-sealing incision. An iridectomy is not routinely suggested because the optic is soft and the optic/haptic junction can act as a gentle hinge. If mechanical blockage of the pupil in the anterior chamber occurred, the iris was pushed forward and the optic, which is soft, would in turn be pushed forward letting the aqueous humor escape through the pupil. In the event of an inflammatory pupil blockage, mydriatic therapy would be proposed first; and if that failed, an iridectomy with the YAG laser was done. At the end of surgery, 500 mg of *DIAMOX®* is systematically administered intravenously and a tablet of 250 mg DIAMOX is also prescribed on the first night after surgery. A one-month antibiotic steroid eye-drop treatment is prescribed postoperatively.

Anatomical Exclusion Criteria

Only patients with normal anterior segments, normal endothelium cell counts, without ocular hypertonia or associated pathologies are considered. It is essential to have a clear crystalline lens and a normal macula.

Choice of Implant

To avoid rotation, the implant is placed along the axis of the anterior chamber's biggest diameter, which, in general, is the vertical diameter. If, for instance, the vertical diameter is the bigger diameter and the implant is placed on the horizontal diameter, this will lead to instability and a risk of the implant rotating. If the implant is well placed on the largest axis, there is no longer any risk of rotation.

Power of the Implant

Choice of the IOL optical power was based on distant refraction according to the Holladay formula.[2] The IOL comes in powers between –5.00 D and +5.00 D. A single addition is available with this model (+2.50 D). All hyperopes between the age of 50 and 60 can be corrected in this way, knowing that the younger subjects will be slightly overcorrected and the older subjects slightly undercorrected. This under- or over-correction has no incidence on everyday life.

Any corneal astigmatism, which alters the quality of the IOL, must be corrected beforehand either with laser or LASIK in order to make the most of this multifocal implant.

RESULTS

Our initial study concerned 55 eyes of 33 patients: 21 women, 12 men, 29 right eyes, 26 left eyes. Preoperative refraction was between –5.00 D and +5.00 D. There were 9 myopic eyes and 46 emmetropic or hyperopic eyes. The anterior chamber was over 3.1 mm in almost all of the cases and the endothelial cell density equal to or above 2,000 C/mm^2. Average age of patients was 54 ± 5.4 years (ranges between 45 and 70 years). The average follow-up was 42.6 weeks (ranges between 83 and 2 weeks).

Refraction

Mean preoperative refraction is + 1.8 D ± 1.3 D (ranges –2.75 D to + 5.00 D) Postoperative mean refraction is – 0.12 D ± 0.51 D (ranges –1.5 D to 1.25 D). There is, therefore, a very satisfactory precise refractive effect. Without going into detail, the first series of patients (Baikoff 3) for whom we used the Van der Heijde formula,[4] showed a higher rate of myopization than the patients subsequently operated on using the more precise Holladay refractive formula.[2]

On the diagrams showing the evolution of the results after one-year follow-up, refraction remains stable (Fig. 6.6).

Distant Visual Acuity

Uncorrected preoperative visual acuity was 0.41 ± 0.29 (decimal scale), and postoperative uncorrected visual acuity (UCVA) was 0.78 ± 0.20 (decimal scale). This uncorrected visual acuity (UCVA) result is equivalent to the other refractive surgery techniques where the mean result is around 0.8.[5-7] Preoperative best-corrected visual acuity is 0.98 ± 0.02 and postoperatively best-

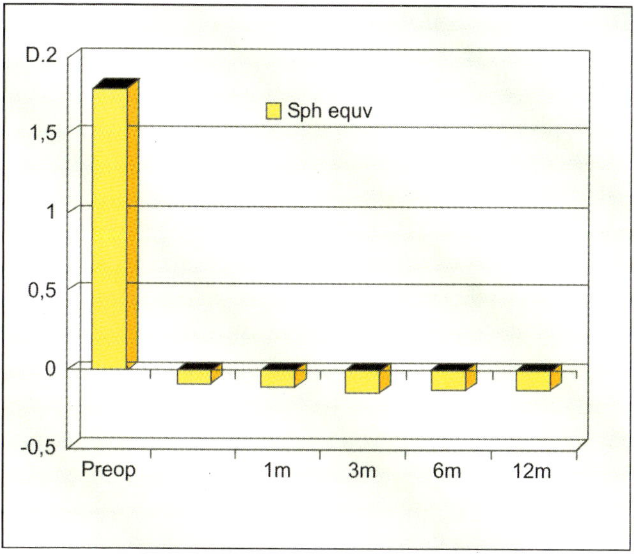

Fig. 6.6: Evolution of postoperative refraction. Stability at 12 months (*Courtesy:* Elsevier)

corrected visual acuity drops to 0.92 ± 0.09. This loss of visual acuity is the result of a drop in contrast sensitivity due to the multifocal lens. It is a well-known fact that multifocal lenses reduce image lighting, decreasing contrast sensitivity and BCVA. This has been observed in pseudophakic IOLS.[8]

Near Visual Acuity

Before surgery, near BCVA is PARINAUD 2.03 + 0.1. Postoperative UCVA is PARINAUD 2.3 ± 0.6 (ranges 2 to 3).

Efficacy and Safety Ratio

The optical and refractive target was obtained, as distant UCVA was satisfactory with a 94 percent safety ratio (postoperative BCVA/preoperative BCVA) and an 80 percent efficacy ratio (postoperative UCVA/ preoperative BCVA). These results were slightly below those that we normally observe with refractive implants where the two factors are respectively between 120 and 140 percent and around 100 percent.[9-12] Finally, UCVA was satisfactory in most cases as 84 percent of eyes operated on obtained 0.6 or better for distant vision and PARINAUD 3 or better for near vision both without correction. These figures correspond to a normally demanding population leading normal everyday lives.

ANATOMICAL RESULTS—INCIDENTS AND COMPLICATIONS

Loss of Visual Acuity

One patient showed a 3-line loss of BCVA three months after surgery of both eyes. Residual myopia existed but despite the correction of this myopia, the patient's visual acuity did not improve. The posterior pole was explored (angiography, OCT, visual field, color vision) and was normal. Three or four months after surgery, visual acuity returned to 1.0. This patient had PRK at a later date to correct her residual myopia with an excellent optical result.

A second patient found her visual acuity reduced to 0.5 and it was impossible to improve after surgery whereas preoperatively she had 0.8. In fact, this 70-year-old patient presented a moderate cataract.

The addition of a multifocal lens in front of a slightly opalescent crystalline lens leads to a very severe drop in visual acuity for two reasons: decrease in light transmission due to the incipient cataract, and a decrease in the lighting of the focused image. In fact, crystalline lens opalescence can reduce retinal illumination by 30 percent and the added effect of a multifocal lens is, therefore, particularly harmful. The implant was removed at the same time as cataract surgery was performed by phacoemulsification using the same 3.2 mm incision. A monofocal implant was inserted into the bag with excellent visual results and a postoperative corrected visual acuity of 1.0.

Loss of Contrast Sensitivity

Loss of contrast sensitivity was not studied objectively, and patients may be sensitive to it after surgery of the first eye as they can compare with the other non-operated eye. A slight grayish sensation is perceived. Once the second eye has been operated on, there is no element of comparison and the discomfort is better accepted. In mesopic vision, that is to say reading at night in dim light conditions, some patients occasionally wear additional glasses.

Reduction of Retinal Illumination

We have seen that the problem with multifocal lenses was a reduction of retinal illumination. One patient suffered from this problem because of a pre-existing crystalline lens pathology (cf supra).

The problems we are faced with concern anatomical predispositions such as senile myosis. A study should be carried out to define the acceptable minimum pupil diameter for this type of implant.

Therefore, multifocal lenses must be contraindicated for patients with slight macular pathologies such as Drüsens or epithelium pigment disorders because they are particularly sensitive to reductions in retinal illumination.

Halos

One of the problems of multifocal lenses is the possibility of parasite optical side effects. We have mentioned before that multifocal lenses reduce contrast sensitivity, however, they also produce halos that are particularly disturbing in night vision. Eighteen percent of eyes and 24 percent of patients complained of halos, but these had no incidence on night driving except in two patients out of 33 (6%).

This high percentage of complaints concerning halos disappears in time because the brain adapts to this inconvenience. In the end, very few patients complained of this discomfort and in time none of them requested change or removal of the implant for this particular reason. Thanks to the Visante™ OCT pupil ovalizations have almost disappeared as the size of the implant is now correctly adapted to the largest axis which is generally the vertical one.

Pupil Ovalization

Ten percent of slight pupil ovalizations showed up under the slit-lamp's intensive light. There were fewer under normal lighting. Generally, pupil ovalizations are the result of oversizing the implant.

Cataract

No implant-induced cataracts have been observed in this study to date.

Ocular Hypertonia

No ocular hypertonia induced by the implant has been observed in this series to date.

Endothelium

After a year, mean endothelial cell loss is below 5 percent. The results meet the FDA's guidelines (Fig. 6.7).

Explantations

Four explantations were carried out on patients who were disappointed with the results. One patient had excellent near and distant vision, 1.0 (decimal scale)

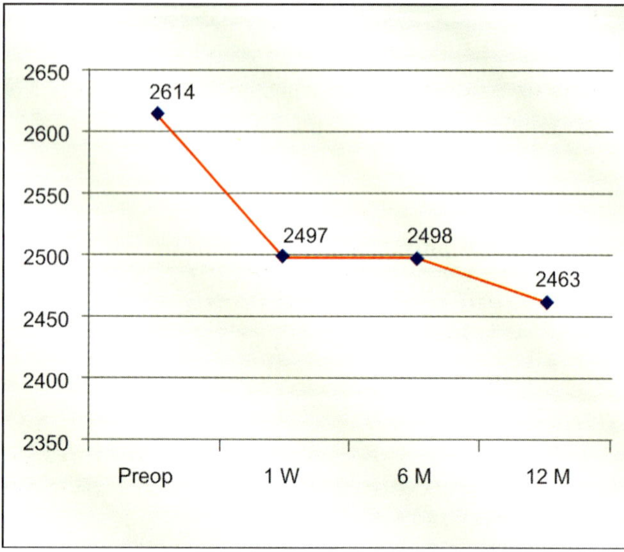

Fig. 6.7: Evolution of corneal endothelium at 1 year (*Courtesy:* Elsevier)

and PARINAUD 2 but was not satisfied with the intermediate vision. He, therefore, requested that the implant be removed.

Two explantations were suggested because of insufficient visual results (cf. supra patient with cataract). One was due to unsolvable postoperative diplopia. In both cases, they recuperated their initial visual status.

Optical defects are inevitable with multifocal lenses, therefore, patient selection must be very strict. Patients too demanding and who think that they will recuperate the vision they had at the age of 20 must be excluded; and before surgery, it is essential to provide precise information concerning the risks and drawbacks of this procedure.

SUMMARY

Since this preliminary study, we have continued to use this technique and to continue rigorous patient selection. The results are confirmed and more than 80 percent of the patients have a distant UCVA over 0.6 D and PARINAUD 3 or better for near vision also uncorrected. This means all the patients lead normal lives without glasses in diurnal conditions; only a few (less than 10%) need them in mesopic conditions, for instance, to read at home in the evenings. In this series, everyday acts are done without glasses. Halos are generally well tolerated and the loss of contrast sensitivity is unavoidable. This technique can, therefore, be proposed but very strict inclusion criteria must be taken into account with regards to anatomy and psychology. This procedure can only be offered to patients with an anterior chamber depth equal to or above 3.0 mm, with an open angle, with a healthy endothelium and without anterior segment or retinal disorders (Fig. 6.8). Any astigmatism must be corrected either before or after implantation. Patients that are too demanding must be excluded as well as patients who, for professional reasons, have to drive at night. The

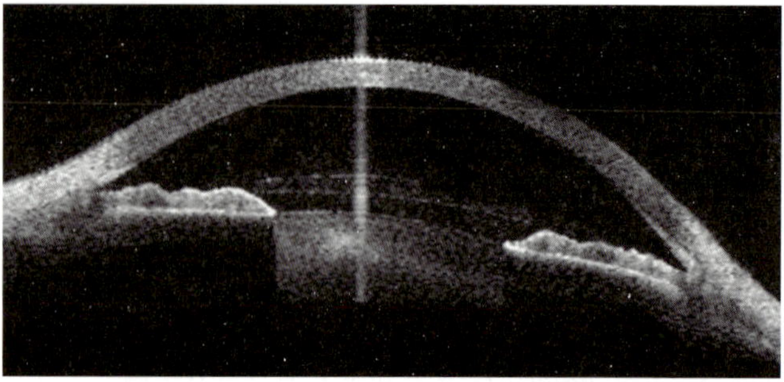

Fig. 6.8: Aspect of a Newlife presbyopic IOL with the AC OCT (*Courtesy:* Elsevier)

interest of phakic implants is their reversibility; in our series, we had no persistent pupillary ovalization after explantation. In certain cases, a mono correction is possible on an emmetropic subject by placing an implant in the dominated eye only. If the result is satisfactory, surgery can be limited to just one eye, and surgery of the other eye proposed only if the patient wishes it. Experience has shown us that patients who had postoperative slightly hypermetropic refraction were more satisfied than patients slightly myopic. This had already been proved with multifocal pseudophakic implants (Steinert).[13] However, to obtain a satisfied patient, it is important to explain that the correction of presbyopia with this multifocal implant for phakic eyes is a compromise between an excellent preoperative vision with glasses and a good postoperative vision without glasses.

REFERENCES

1. Lindström R. Correction of presbyopia with intraocular and intracorneal lenses Binkhorst Lecture. American Society of Refractive and Cataract Meeting. San Francisco California, 12 April 2003.
2. Holladay JT. Refractive power calculations for intraocular lenses in the phakic eye. Am J Ophthalmol 1993;15,116(1): 63-66.
3. Baïkoff G. Presbyopic phakic intraocular lenses. In Agarwal A (Ed): Presbyopia: A Surgical Textbook: Thorofare NJ: Slack Inc 2002;225-28.
4. Fechner PU ,Van Der Heijde GL , Worst JGF. The correction of myopia by lens implantation into phakic eyes. Am J Ophthalmol 1989;107:659-63.
5. Sawelson H, Marks RG. Ten years refractive and visual results of radial keratotomy. Ophthalmology 1995; 102:1892-1901.
6. Hersh PS, Stulting RD, Steinert RF, et al. Results of phase III Excimer laser photorefractive keratectomy for myopia. The Summit PRK study group. Ophthalmology 1997;104: 1535-53.
7. Davidorf JM, Zaldivar R, Oscherow S. Results and complications of laser *in situ* keratomileusis by experienced surgeons. J Refract Surg 1998;14:114-22.
8. Monte–Mico R, Alio J. Distance and near contrast sensitivity function after multifocal intraocular lens implantation. J Cataract Refract Surg 2003;29(4):703-11.
9. Perez-Santoja JJ, Alio JL, Jimenez–Alfaro I, Zato MA. Surgical correction of severe myopia with an angle supported phakic intraocular lens. J Cataract Refract Surg 2000;26(9):1288-302.
10. Baïkoff G, Arne JL, Bokobza Y, et al. Angle fixated anterior chamber phakic intraocular lens for myopia of –7 to –9 diopters. J Refract Surg 1998;14:282-93.
11. Menezo JL, Avino JA, Cisneros A, et al. Iris claw phakic intraocular lens for high myopia. J Refract Surg 1997;13: 545-55.

12. Zaldivar R, Oscherow S, Ricur G. Implantable contact lens. In: Clear Corneal Lens Surgery. Thorofare, NJ: Slack Inc 1999;287-324.
13. Steinert RF, Aker BL, Trentacost DJ, et al. A prospective study of the AMO-Array zonal progressive multifocal silicone intraocular lens and a monofocal intraocular lens. Ophthalmology 1999;106:1243-45.

CHAPTER 7

Multifocal Refractive Lenses for Presbyopia

Ashok Garg (India)

INTRODUCTION

Multifocal Refractive Lens Technology offers a greater benefits for the patients. The elimination of a presbyopic condition and restoration of normal vision by simulating accommodation greatly enhances the quality of the life for most of the patients. The advantages of astigmatically neutral clear corneal surgery have allowed for increased utilization for multifocal technology in lens based refractive surgery. It will allow surgeons to offer multifocal technology to their patients with better visual outcome.

The loss of accommodative ability following cataract surgery has been overcome to an extent by the development of intraocular lenses with multifocal optics.[1-3] The different types of multifocal IOLs are the diffractive type, which provides distance vision by refraction and near vision by diffraction from a series of phase controlled concentric slopes on the posterior lens surface, the refractive aspheric type and the two or three zone refractive type.[4] The last mentioned IOL design is now obsolete because of extensive side effects that affected the quality of vision and will not be discussed further in this discussion.

Another option available nowadays for the correction of postoperative presbyopia is accommodative IOLs. These lenses are based on the focus shift principle, which involves movement of the IOL within the capsular sac. The hinged design allows the lens to move forward as the eye attempts to focus on near objects restoring some amount of accommodative function. Accommodative lenses have plate haptics which when placed into the capsular bag, vaults anteriorly upon contraction of the ciliary body, akin to the natural physiology of the crystalline lens and the ciliary body. The extensive use of multifocal intraocular lens has been limited till now because of certain inherent problems associated with these IOLs in the form of decreased contrast sensitivity and severe visual symptoms like discomfort at night, halos, and glare. The newer designs incorporating aspheric optics and asymmetrical light distribution, decreases many of these problems, ensures satisfactory intermediate vision, and thus offers better quality of vision.

MULTIFOCAL IOLs

Multifocal IOLs work on the principles of simultaneous imaging of two optical systems at least 3 D apart. The brain interprets the two images as separate images, selects the more focused image and suppresses the other. The optical performance of multifocal intraocular lenses has improved over the last few years. The clinical results have also improved due to the application of the astigmatically neutral small incision surgery. However, the system-inherent characteristics of multifocal lenses, namely a severe loss in the contrast visual acuity as well as disturbing scattering of light have persisted and form a limiting factor for larger-scale standard application of these IOLs. The reason for this is that in the older variety of refractive-diffractive lenses, the light distribution in both the main foci being 50 percent each, resulted in reduced light intensity and contrast visual acuity as compared to monofocal lenses. Furthermore, the dependence of contrast visual acuity on the pupil width and perfect centration of the IOL resulted in accentuation of symptoms of reduced contrast, halos and glare.

The different types of multifocal IOLs are:

Diffractive IOLs

The diffractive IOLs provide distance vision by refraction and near vision by using diffraction from series of phase controlled concentric slopes on the posterior lens surface. Since these concentric rings for near and distance are present in the center of the lens itself, decentration of the IOL or the pupillary size does not affect vision. One of the main disadvantages of these IOLs has been the compromise in the resolution of the image when the contrast of the focused image is reduced by the out of focus images due to incomplete cortical suppression.

Nonfoldable diffractive multifocal IOLs are available by Pharmacia in both PMMA (CeeOn 811E) and silicone (Z9000M), and by Alcon in acrylic (MA60D3).

With the increasing need to adapt multifocal IOLs to smaller incisions, diffractive multifocal IOLs are available now as foldable lenses (AcriTec GmbH,

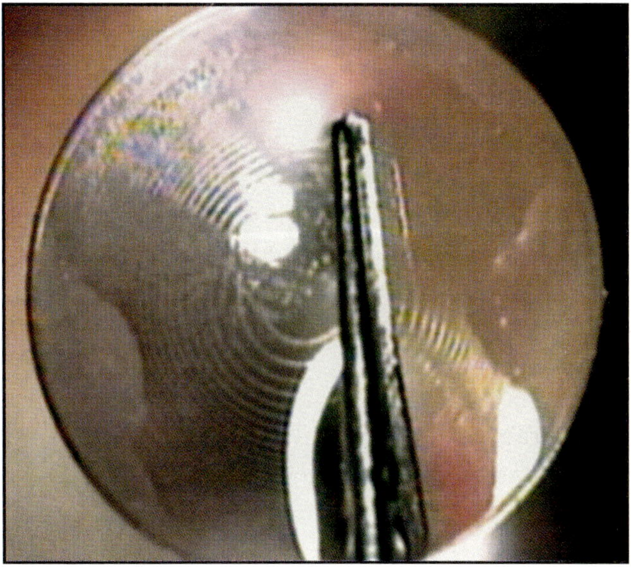

Fig. 7.1: Diffractive multifocal IOL

Munich). This is a 3-piece foldable silicone IOL with a 6 mm optic. It is biconvex, aspheric with Fresnel zones available from +0.00 D to +40.00 D which has been used with good results in terms of patient satisfaction. These bifocal intraocular lenses are characterized by an asymmetrical light distribution. The dominant eye is implanted with a bifocal lens with light distribution of 70 percent for the far focus and 30 percent for the near focus. The accompanying eye receives an intraocular lens with a light distribution of 70 percent for the near focus and 30 percent for the far focus. As a result, with planned bilateral implantation of the IOL, considerable

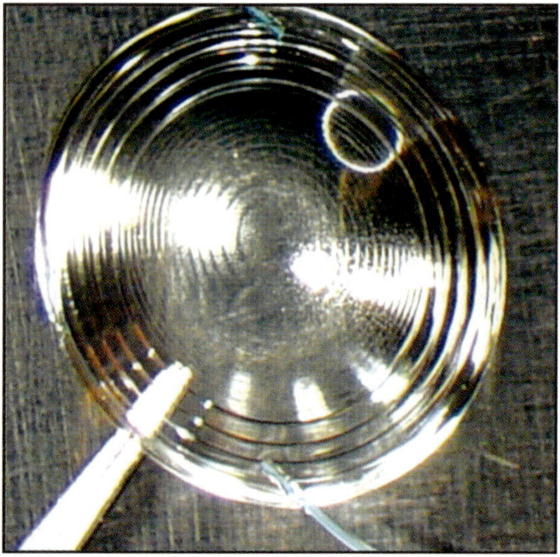

Fig. 7.2: Foldable bifocal AcriTec Twin Set 737 D / 733 D

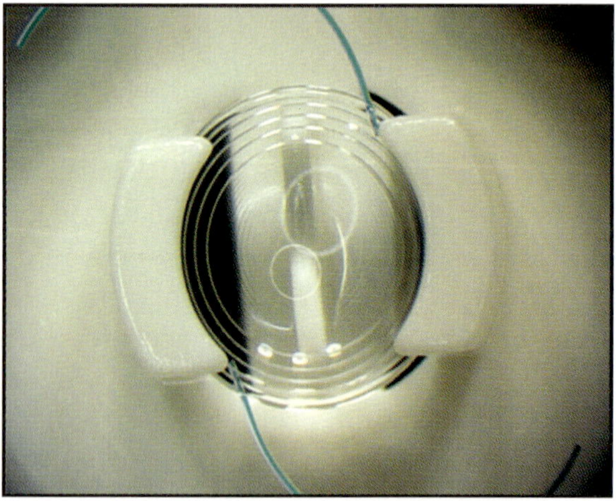

Fig. 7.3: A 38 D bifocal foldable AcriTec IOL showing Fresnel zones

improvement of the contrast can be achieved. The contrast visual acuity is such a case is only reduced by a factor of 1.4 as compared to a factor of almost 2 with multifocal lenses with symmetrical bifocal intraocular lenses. These lenses are reported to have extremely low secondary cataract rate, hold a firm and steady position in the capsular bag, demonstrate no vaulting, bending or decentration of the IOL. The smaller incision is more stable, shows lesser astigmatism and faster wound healing.

Refractive Multifocal IOL Implant

The Array multifocal IOL implant is a silicone IOL of the refractive multifocal type. This lens incorporates in

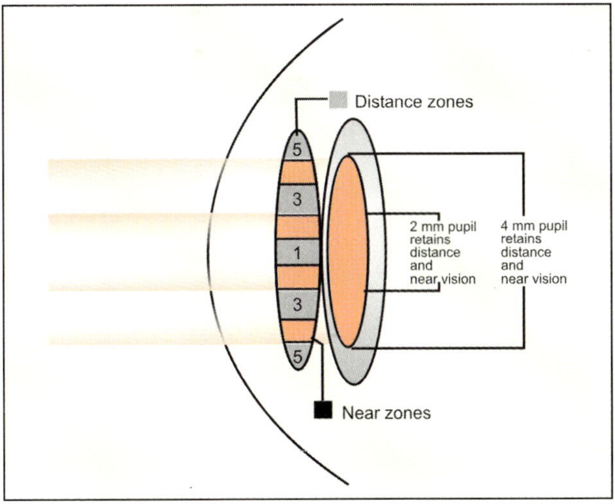

Fig. 7.4: Optics of the Refractive Array Multifocal IOL

its surface concentric rings of varying power around a central power for distance. This central power is dominant over the peripheral "near" power. 50 percent of the IOL is dedicated to distance vision, 36 percent to near vision and the remaining 14 percent to intermediate vision. Good contrast sensitivity is maintained in this IOL due to the asymmetric light distribution. A bothersome side effect especially associated with the use of this particular type of IOL is halos around lights especially at night. The reason for the same is not clear. However, this side effect needs to be explained to the patient prior to surgery.

Older Models of Two or Three Zone Refraction Type of IOL

The older models of two or three zone refraction type of IOL as has been used previously are no longer in use because of the subjective deterioration of the quality of vision caused by them in the form of decreased contrast sensitivity, glare, halos, etc. Hence they have not been discussed further in this chapter.

Accommodative IOLs

Certain newer types of IOLs have been developed that take into account the normal physiological interplay of the ciliary body with the crystalline lens (replaced by the capsular bag containing the IOL postoperatively). These accommodative IOLs like the Human Optics Accommodative 1 CU IOL are designed to

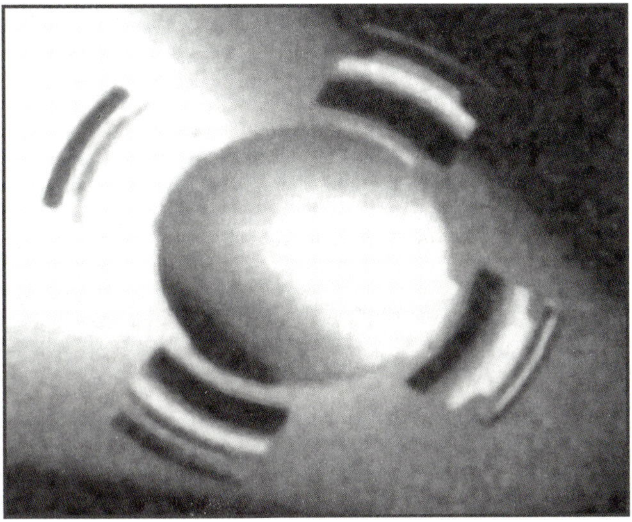

Fig. 7.5: Accommodative IOL

transform the contracting forces of the ciliary muscle into anterior movement of the IOL optic. The pseudophakic accommodation by this method has been measured between 1.3 D to 1.7 D as the lens performs an anterior focus shift of about 0.65 mm.

The principle of these lenses are that when the haptic plates are placed in the capsular bag, the anterior capsule fibroses and applies pressure on the haptics which vault posteriorly such that the optic lies next to the vitreous face. With the contraction of the ciliary muscle and its subsequent pressure on the vitreous face, the optics move forward resulting in pseudophakic accommodation. These lenses are larger lenses available as both non-foldable and foldable IOLs.

Crystalens was the first accommodative IOL available for use in the US. Another accommodating IOL, the AT-45 silicone accommodative intraocular lens is undergoing the initial phases of the FDA trial.

MULTIFOCAL IOLs AND MICROINCISION CATARACT SURGERY

Technology runs forward in leaps and bounds. Starting from the Ridley IOLs to modern day micro-incision cataract surgery IOLs has been a long journey spanning over half a century. As the desire for perfection increases, the unwanted effects of the older procedures, equipments or implants are modified so as to increase the benefits derived from the same procedure, equipment or implants. Sometimes, one technology may advance faster than other complementary technologies. To cite an example, phacoemulsification became a routine procedure for performing cataract extraction much before the advent of foldable IOLs. Thus though the procedure could be performed through a 3 mm incision, the incision had to be increased to a minimum of 5.5 mm to incorporate the IOLs. We have a similar situation again, when cataract extraction can be performed through incisions as small as 1 mm, but the IOL technology is just beginning to explore the possibilities of inserting IOLs through that small an incision and simultaneously maintaining the optical quality of the inserted IOLs. Thus the ongoing research not only has to evaluate the long-term benefits, results and efficacy of these newer IOLs but also the associated technique of its appropriate insertion through a microincision. This includes designs for newer injecting systems that are safe and maintain the quality of the IOL while the insertion is taking place.

Another dream remains the amelioration of post-operative presbyopia. Most new models of multifocal IOLs incorporate special aspherical designs with asymmetrical light distribution that takes into account the spherical aberration of the cornea and the loss of contrast due to symmetrical light distribution in the two foci for distance and near. Due to the rotational symmetry of these new lenses, the image is also independent of the diameter of the pupil. Thus many problems of the yesteryears have been taken care of multifocal IOLs are now available as foldable IOLs and trials are on to assess the long-term results of these newer generation IOLs. These IOLs thus facilitate both, the nondistortion of a small, astigmatically neutral incision and the amelioration of postoperative presbyopia thus simulating or at times bettering the preoperative visual status in the immediate postoperative period. These could be of specific use in the pediatric age group where amblyopia is a major concern. Being able to correct vision for both distance and near would be of immense benefit in these cases.

Pseudoaccommodation has been a feature of many lenses, both silicone and acrylic, that have been used for microincision cataract surgery. This has been hypothesized to be due to the ultrathin thickness of these lenses which aids the normal physiological accommodative response of the capsular bag upon contraction of the ciliary muscle. Longer trials are required to authenticate these hypotheses.

The symbiosis and subsequent syntheses of the newer generation IOLs incorporating larger lenses with accommodative and multifocal optics and the ultra-thin lenses with the quality of pseudoaccommodation for use in microincision cataract surgery remains a dream today. But just as the dreams of yesterday have become realities today in our continuous quest for perfection, there is no reason to think that true accommodative and multifocal IOLs that can be incorporated through a microincision of 1 to 1.5 mm will not become a viable reality tomorrow.

REFERENCES

1. Montes-Mico R, Alió JL. Distance and near contrast sensitivity function after multifocal intraocular lens implantation. J Cataract Refract Surg 2003; 29:703-11.
2. Findl O, Kiss B, Petternel V, Menapace R, Georgopoulos M, et al. Intraocular lens movement caused by ciliary body contraction. J Cataract Refract Surg 2003; 29:669-76.
3. Kuchle M, Seitz B, Langenbucher A, Gusek-Schneider GC, Martus P, et al. The Erlangen Accommodative Intraocular Lens Study Group. Comparison of 6 months results of implantation of the 1 CU accommodative intraocular lenses with conventional intraocular lenses. Ophthalmology 2004; 111:825-34.
4. Humming JS, Slade SG, Chayet A, AT-45 Study Group. Clinical evaluation of the model AT-45 silicone accommodating intraocular lens: Results of feasibility and the initial phase of the FDA Clinical Trial. Ophthalmology 2001;108: 2005-10.

CHAPTER 8

Presbyopic LASIK—A New Hope

Amar Agarwal, Athiya Agarwal, Sunita Agarwal,
Ashok Garg (India), Guillermo Avalos Urzua (Mexico)

INTRODUCTION

Presbyopia, is the final frontier for an ophthalmologist. In the 21st century the latest developments, which are taking place, are in the field of presbyopia. In presbyopia, the nearest point that can be focused gradually recedes, leading to the need for optical prosthesis for close work such as reading and eventually even for focus in the middle distance.

PREVIOUS EXCIMER LASER TECHNIQUES

Presbyopic photorefractive keratectomy (PRK) has been tried. In this using the excimer laser, a mask consisting of a mobile diaphragm formed by two blunt blades was used to ablate a 10 to 17 micron deep semilunar-shaped zone immediately below the papillary center, steepening the corneal curvature in that area.

Monofocal vision with LASIK has also been tried to solve the problem of presbyopia. The goal in such cases is to make the patient anisometropic. In this one eye is used for distance vision and the other for near-vision. This is obviously not indicated in all subjects. The residual consequences are partial loss of stereopsis, asthenopia, headache, aneisokonia and decreased binocularity.

HISTORY

Guillermo Avalos[1,2] started the idea of presbyopic LASIK. This is called the PARM technique. He held a live surgical conference in Mexico where he had invited the Agarwals to perform phakonit and the no-anesthesia cataract surgery technique. There, he discussed with them the idea of presbyopic LASIK and when they came back they started the technique.

PRINCIPLE

The objective is to allow the patient to focus on near objects while retaining his ability to focus on far objects, taking into account the refractive error of the eye when the treatment is performed. With this LASIK technique the corneal curvature is modified, creating a bilateral multifocal cornea in the treated optical zone. A combination of hyperopic and myopic LASIK is done aiming to make a multifocal cornea. We determine if the eye is presbyopic plano, presbyopic with spherical hyperopia or presbyopia with spherical myopia. These may also have astigmatism in which case the astigmatism is treated at the same time.

PROLATE AND OBLATE CORNEA

It is important for us to understand a prolate and oblate cornea before we progress further on the technique of presbyopic LASIK. The shape of spheroid (a conoidal surface of revolution) is qualitatively prolate or oblate, depending on whether it is stretched or flattened in its axial dimension. In a prolate cornea the meridional curvature decreases from pole to equator and in an oblate cornea the meridional curvature continually increases. The optical surfaces of the normal human eye both cornea and lens is prolate. This shape has an optical advantage in that spherical aberration can be avoided. Following LASIK the prolateness of the anterior cornea reduces but is insufficient to eliminate its spherical aberration. Thus, one should remember the normal cornea is prolate. When myopic LASIK is done the cornea becomes oblate. When hyperopic LASIK is done the cornea becomes prolate.

Every patient treated with an excimer laser is left with an oblate or prolate shaped cornea depending upon the myopia or hyperopia of the patient. The approach to improve visual quality after LASIK is to apply geometric optics and use the patient's refraction, precise preoperative corneal height data and optimal postoperative anterior corneal shape in order to have a customized prolate shape treatment.

TECHNIQUE

First of all a superficial corneal flap is created with the microkeratome. The corneal flap performed with the microkeratome must be between 8.5 to 9.5 mm in order to have an available corneal surface for treatment of at least 8 mm. In this way, the laser beam does not touch the hinge of the flap. In India the Bausch and Lomb LASIK machine is used and in Mexico the Apollo machine is used. Once the flap has been created a hyperopic ablation in an optical zone of 5 mm is done

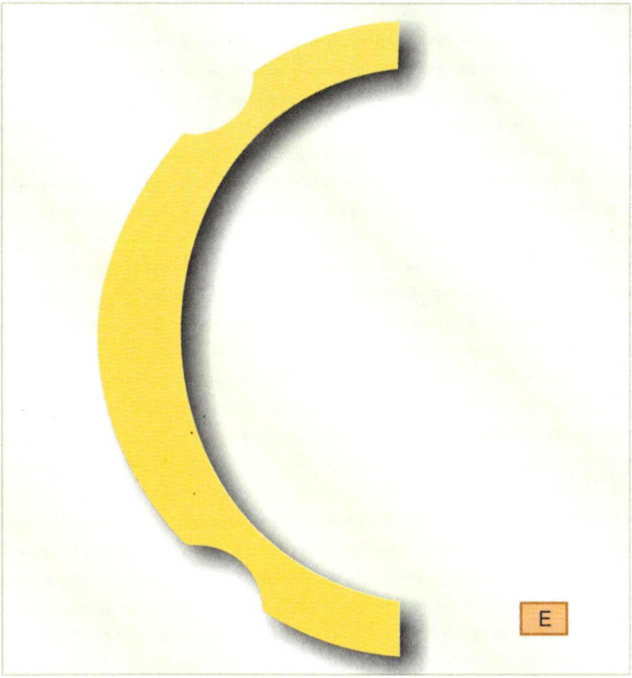

Fig. 8.1: Hyperopic LASIK done on the cornea. Myopic prolate cornea produced

(Fig. 8.1). The treated cornea now has a steepness section. The cornea is thus myopic, prolate. This allows the eye to focus in a range that includes near vision but excludes far vision.

With this myopic-shaped cornea, one now selects a smaller area of the central cornea that is concentric with the previous worked area. The size of the area is a 4 mm optical zone. A myopic LASIK is now done with the 4 mm optical zone (Fig. 8.2). The resulting cornea

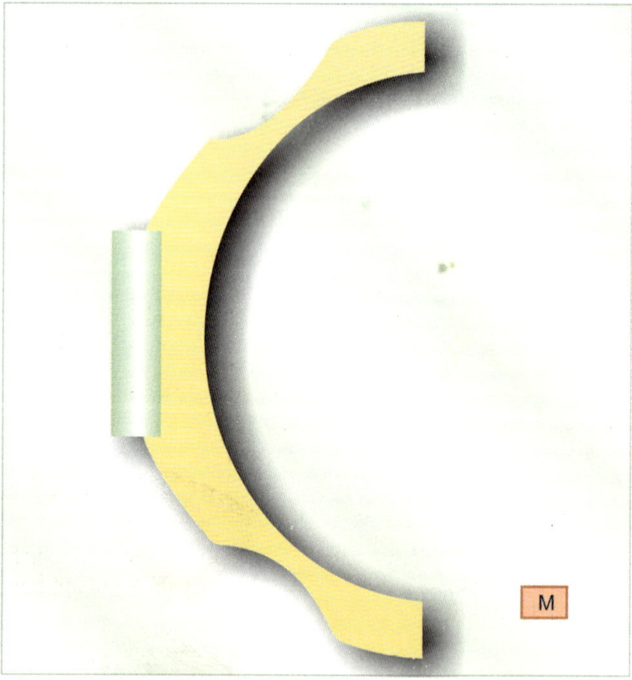

Fig. 8.2: Myopic LASIK done. Myopic ablation of 4 mm optical zone performed to create a central oblate cornea

now has a central area (oblate) that is configured for the eye to focus on far objects and a ring-shaped area that allows the eye to focus on near objects (Fig. 8.3). The flap is now cleaned and replaced back in position.

KERATOMETRY AND PACHYMETRY

Pachymetry is not important for this procedure. The preoperative keratometry reading is extremely

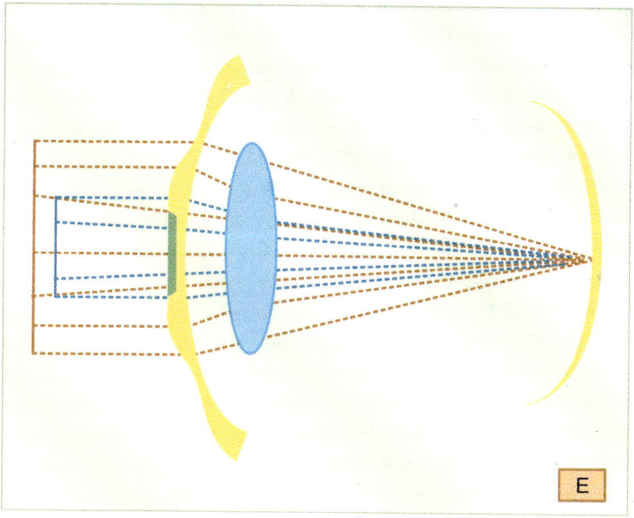

Fig. 8.3: Schematic diagram of a presbyopic cornea in which hyperopic and myopic LASIK has been done. The patient can thus focus for near and distance

important. The postoperative keratometer reading should not exceed 48 D. The keratometer reading should be taken from topography and not from a manual keratometer machine. For each hypermetropic diopter corrected, the corneal curvature increases in 0.89 keratometric diopters as an average. It is recommended to treat patients with keratometry in the range between 41 to 43 D to obtain postoperative curves under 48 D. If the cornea is more than 48 D, it produces undesired optical alterations like glare, halos, decreased visual acuity and decreased contrast sensitivity. The preoperative and postoperative keratometer readings should be nearly the same for the patient to be comfortable.

ASTIGMATISM

If astigmatism is present, it is recommended to use as a limit 2.5 D. One should also remember there is an induced astigmatism of 0.5 to 0.75 D created by the corneal shape after the surgery and this can decrease one or two lines of uncorrected visual acuity.

Plano Examples

Now let us look at treating presbyopic patients who are basically plano for distance.

Example 1

Let us take a patient who is plano for distance and is 20/20. For near on addition of + 2 D the patient is J1. The preoperative keratometer let us say is 41 D.

There are three steps in the presbyopic LASIK treatment.

1 Step—For distance—No treatment is required as the patient is plano 20/20.

2 Step—For near—Hyperopic LASIK is done of + 2 D. A 5 mm optical zone is taken. We have already mentioned that each diopter of hyperopia corrected changes the corneal curvature by 0.89 D, which is approximately 1 D. So the keratometer changes from 41 to 43 D (approximately).

3 Step—Myopic LASIK of –1 D with a 4 mm optical zone. So keratometer now becomes 42 D.

Regression occurs for hyperopia treatment to about 1 D, so we have done myopic ablation of –1 and not –2 D. The preoperative keratometer reading was 41 D and postoperative keratometer reading is 42 D, which is nearly the same.

Hyperopic Examples

Now let us look at presbyopic LASIK being performed in a hyperopic eye.

Example 2

Let us take a patient who is hyperopic for distance and is 20/20 with + 1 D. For near on addition of + 3 D the patient is J1. The preoperative keratometer let us say is 42 D.

There are three steps in the presbyopic LASIK treatment.

1 Step—For distance—Hyperopic LASIK is done of + 1 D with a 5 mm optical zone. So keratometer changes from 42 D to 43 D.

2 Step—For near—Hyperopic LASIK is done of + 3 D. A 5 mm optical zone is taken. We have already mentioned that each diopter of hyperopia corrected changes the corneal curvature by 0.89 D, which is approximately 1 D. So the keratometer changes from 43 to 46 D (approximately).

3 Step—Myopic LASIK of –2 D with a 4 mm optical zone. So keratometer now becomes 44 D.

Regression occurs for hyperopia treatment to about 1 D, so we have done myopic ablation of –2 and not –3 D. The preoperative keratometer reading was 42 D but after making the patient plano it is 43 D. The postoperative keratometer reading is 44 D, which is nearly the same.

Though we have to correct totally 4 D for hypermetropia we take it in two steps. One should not do it in one step as that much hyperopia corrected in one step makes the central cornea too steep to perform the myopic ablation.

Example 3

Let us take a patient who is hyperopic for distance and is 20/20 with + 3 D. For near on addition of + 3 D the patient is J1. The preoperative keratometer let us say is 44 D.

The preoperative keratometer reading is 44 D and we have to correct 3 D for distance and 3 D for near. So if we do presbyopic LASIK we will make the keratometer reading 50 D. So, one should not treat such patients with presbyopia LASIK.

Myopic Example

Now let us look at myopic patients.

Example 4

Let us take a patient who is myopic for distance and is 20/20 with –2 D. For near on addition of + 2 D the patient is J1. This means the patient is plano for near. The preoperative keratometer let us say is 43 D.

There are three steps in the presbyopic LASIK treatment.

1 Step—For distance- Patient is myopic so no treatment is required.

2 Step—For near- Hyperopic LASIK is done of + 2 D. A 5 mm optical zone is taken. We have already mentioned that each diopter of hyperopia corrected changes the corneal curvature by 0.89 D, which is approximately 1 D. So the keratometer changes from 43 to 45 D (approximately).

3 Step—Myopic LASIK of –3 D with a 4 mm optical zone. So keratometer now becomes 42 D.

Regression occurs for hyperopia treatment to about 1 D, so we have done myopic ablation of –3 and not –4 D. The preoperative keratometer reading was 43 D but patient was myopic by 2 D, so actually the keratometer reading should be 41 D. The postoperative keratometer reading is 42 D, which is nearly the same.

We did myopic ablation of 3 D, as patient is myopic of 2 D and presbyopic of 2 D. Regression factor taken is 1 D.

SUMMARY

This idea of presbyopic LASIK is not the end of it all. This technique needs further improvizations to become the technique of choice for one and all.

REFERENCES

1. Guillermo Avalos. Presbyopic LASIK—the PARM technique in Amar Agarwal's Presbyopia: A surgical Textbook. Slack Inc, USA, 2002.
2. Agarwal T et al. Presbyopic LASIK—the Agarwal Technique in Amar Agarwal's Presbyopia: A Surgical Textbook. Slack Inc, USA, 2002.

CHAPTER 9

Presbyopia Treatment with LASIK: PARM (Presbyopia Avalos Rozakis Method)

Guillermo Avalos Urzua (Mexico)

INTRODUCTION

Presbyopia is the age-related normal process where accommodation is lost and the eye is no longer capable to comfortably sustain the accommodation necessary for clear near vision. It is a fact that the range of accommodative amplitude decreases with increasing age, such that the nearest point that can be focused gradually recedes, leading (in humans, at least) to the need for optical prostheses for close work such as reading and, eventually, even for focus in the middle distance (Figs 9.1 and 9.2).

It is the most frequent eye problem in the world, since 40 percent of the population is presbyopic. In Latin America there are 115 millions of presbyopic, and every year this number increases up to three millions;

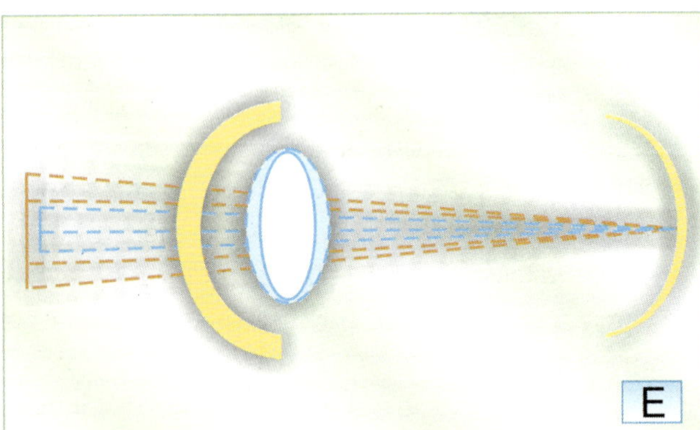

Fig. 9.1: Normal accommodation of the lens for near and distance vision, clear focus over retina

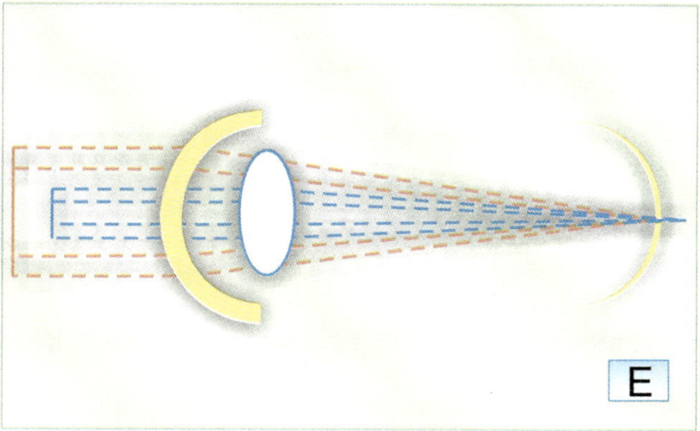

Fig. 9.2: Loss of accommodation of the lens for near vision, clear focus just for distance

it is said that in 2010 there are going to be almost 145 millions. Even though it is not a legal blindness cause, the cost from this problem in productivity loss is high in USA. In presbyopia the nearest point that can be focused gradually recedes, leading to the need for optical prostheses for close work such as reading and, eventually, even for focus in the middle distance. For emmetropic persons, presbyopia seems to appear practically overnight when they reach their mid 40s. However, the loss of near focus is actually progressive over a person's lifetime, whether he or she is emmetropic, myopic, or hyperopic, and the age at which a person requires assistance for near focus will depend in large part on his or her refractive error (Fig. 9.3).

In order to understand more the geometry of the cornea and its topography is necessary to review some

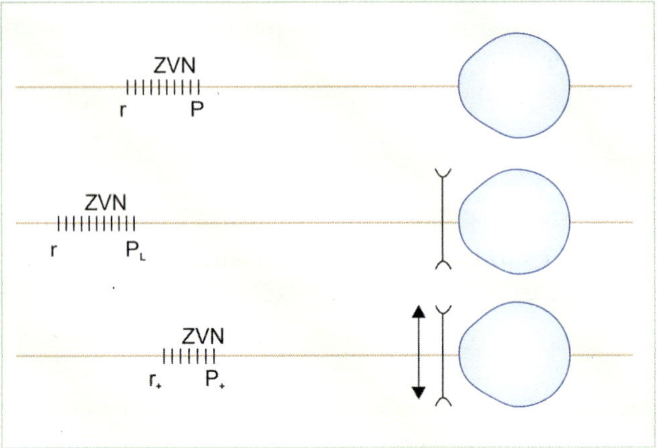

Fig. 9.3: Clear visual zones in an emmetropic eye (a), neutralizing (b) and with add correction (c)

concepts. First, an axis-based curvature is any directed curvature measured relative to the current view axis. Several axis-based curvatures are used (or at least defined) in corneal topography. Axial and meridional curvatures are oblique and measured in meridional planes, while radial and transverse curvatures are normal curvatures. All axis-based curvatures have axial artifacts.

Axial curvature is the radial average of meridional curvature from the view-axis to the surface point of interest, or equivalently, it is the reciprocal of the meridian-normal distance from a surface point to the view axis. As axial curvature was the rawest form of mapped placido data, it formed the original and still the most popular corneal topography map. When compared to meridional maps, axial features are smoother and larger in extent, which is a direct consequence of the radial smoothing via averaging.

Meridional curvature is local surface curvature measured in meridional planes. It is generally oblique (not normal), except for asymmetric surfaces.

Radial curvature is a local surface curvature measured in radial planes, which are surface normal planes lying perpendicular to traverse planes.

Transverse curvature is a local surface curvature measured in transverse planes, which are surface normal planes lying perpendicular to meridional planes. Historically, transverse curvature is also known as sagittal curvature.

The shape of spheroid (a conoidal surface of revolution) is qualitatively prolate or oblate, depending on whether it is stretched or flattened in its axial dimension. More precisely, a surface of revolution is prolate if its meridional curvature decreases from pole to equator, and oblate if it continually increases. The sphere stands between the prolate and oblate continua of surfaces.

The optical surfaces of the normal human eye, both cornea and lens are prolate. This shape has an optical advantage, in that spherical aberration (the primary aberration of a spherical surface) can be avoided. The prolateness of the anterior cornea reduces but is insufficient to eliminate its spherical aberration.

Every patient treated with an excimer laser is left with an oblate-shaped cornea. The approach to improve visual quality after LASIK is to apply geometric optics and use the patient's refraction, precise preoperative corneal height data and optimal postoperative anterior corneal shape, in order to have a customized prolate shape treatment.

PARM* relates to an apparatus and technique for altering the shape of the cornea to have two concentric vision zones that help a presbyopic patient to focus on near items and far items. The objective is to allow the patient to focus on near objects while retaining his ability to focus on far objects, taking into account the refractive error of the eye when the treatment is performed. With this LASIK technique the corneal curvature is modified, creating a bilateral bifocal cornea. The preoperatively corneal curvature is the main factor to consider in this type of corrective method. Pachymetry is not fundamental for this treatment, but it is the focusing ability of the eye measured by refractometry. The doctor performing the method next determines an appropriate level of correction that must be applied to cornea to allow eye to focus on objects in range. Having these measurements, we will determine if the eye is presbyopic plano, presbyopic with spherical hyperopia, or presbyopic with spherical myopia. It may also be determined that any of these three conditions is combined with astigmatism, in these cases astigmatism is treated at the same time.

If we have a presbyopic patient of +2.00 D, but plano meaning that no correction is needed to achieve

20/20 vision other than the correction for the presbyopic condition, a central area of the cornea is selected to perform the initial treatment. In the present context, this central area is 6 mm optical zone. A flap is then done and the initial treatment is performed by eroding the tissue with a laser beam. The boundaries and definition of area are determined using a difference of sphere algorithm mathematically, developed for PARM*, defined in a way that laser can be controlled to remove this tissue.

The preferred treatment for removing area is to sculpt cornea with four sequential collapsing crescent-shaped laser beams. It begins with a half circle-shaped laser applied to the left half area. The intensity of laser and the amount of time it is applied to the central area, are determined by a controller designed for PARM*, that analyzes the zone and determines the time and intensity requires for the laser to remove the tissue. The size of laser gradually collapses until it disappears in the direction from the center corneal area to its edge; the right side corneal area is then treated. Once left and right corneal areas are treated, the doctor changes the laser configuration and treats the top and the bottom sections of the central corneal area (Figs 9.4A and B).

Treated cornea now has a steepness section (the cornea is thus myopic, prolate) that allows eye to focus in range that include near vision, but excludes far vision. With this myopic-shaped cornea, the doctor now selects a smaller area of the central cornea that is

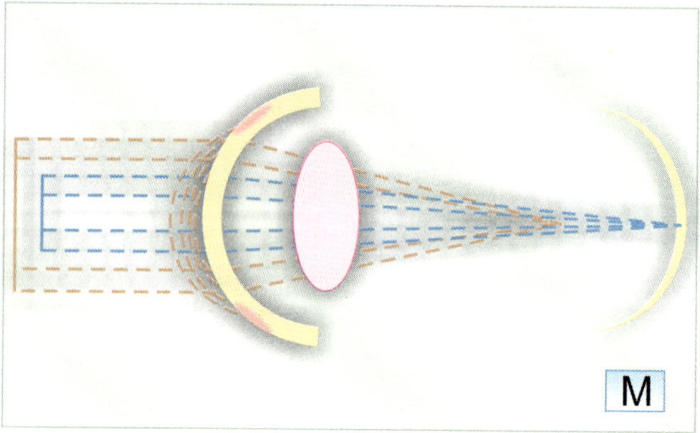

Fig. 9.4A: Treated 6 mm optical zone, the resulting cornea has a peripheral ablation and central steepness. Eye is able to focus just near objects

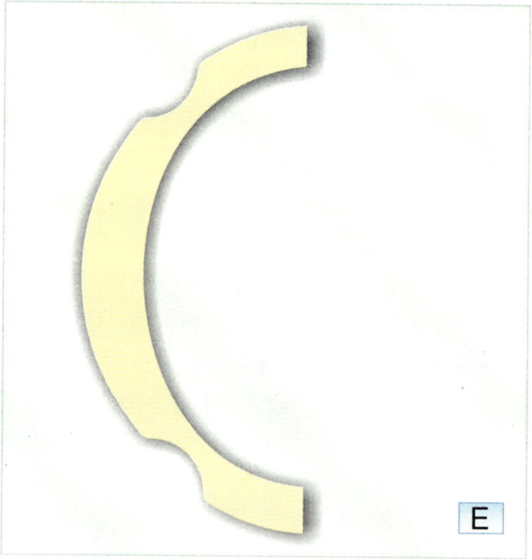

Fig. 9.4B: Ablated 6 mm zone, peripheral ablation and central steepness

concentric with the previous worked area; the size of the area is a 4 mm optical zone. The doctor applies a treatment to this 4 mm zone that allows the cornea to focus on objects far away, thus treating the myopic condition. This treatment is a spherical diopter correction equal to, but negative of the positive correction applied to the 6 mm zone. In this example, a negative 2.00 D correction is performed in the area of 4 mm. The resulting cornea has a central area (oblate) that is configures for the eye to focus on far objects and a ring-shaped area that allows the eye to focus in near objects (Figs 9.5A and B).

Having undergone this treatment, the presbyopic patient can now focus on near and far objects without the use of implants or reading glasses.

When the eye is hyperopic, PARM* is altered to also correct the hyperopia. For instance, the central zone of 6 mm is initially treated with a +2.00 D correction, along with a correction for the hyperopia. For example, in a patient with hyperopia of +3.00 D and presbyopia of +2.00 D, the correction first applied to the central zone of 6 mm is a resulting + 5.00 D spherical correction [(hyperopia + 3.00 D)+ (presbyopia +2.00 D)]; the zone of 4 mm is secondly treated with a –2.00 D correction resulting in the correction of the hyperopia in addition to the presbyopia.

When the eye is myopic, the initial correction area includes a combination of the presbyopic correction with a myopic correction. For example, when the eye is

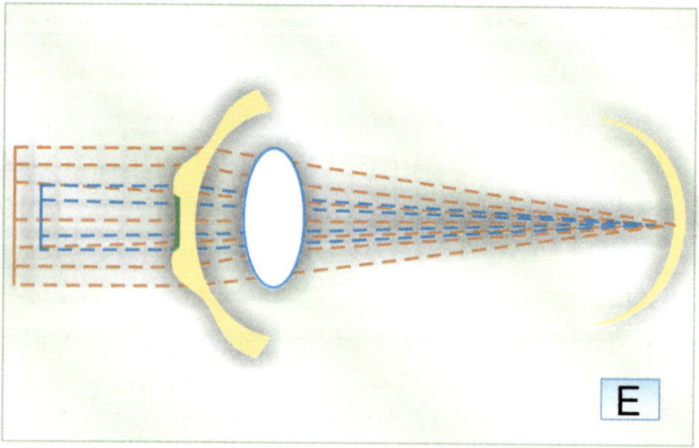

Fig. 9.5A: Treated 4 mm optical zone, the resulting cornea has a flat section that allows eye to focus far objects plus 6 mm ablation that allows eye to focus near

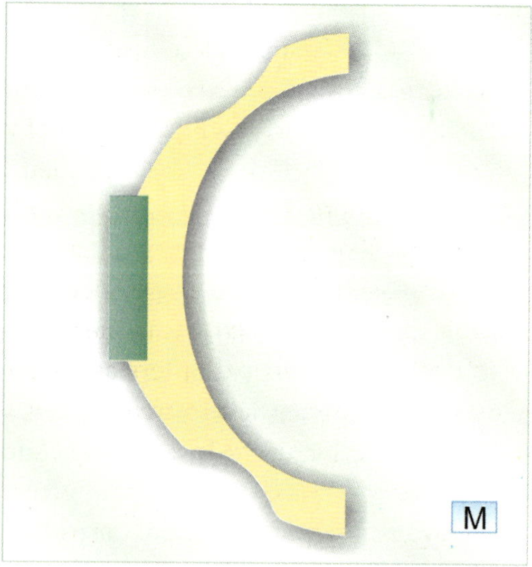

Fig. 9.5B: Ablated 4 mm (green) and 6 mm zone, peripheral ablation and central flatness

–3.00D myopic and +2.00 D presbyopic, the presbyopia correction to central area of 6 mm is a positive 2 D correction; the central area of 4 mm is then treated with a negative 5.00 D spherical diopter correction as suggested by PARM* and determined by combining a negative 3 D spherical from the myopia with a negative 2.00 D spherical correction induced by PARM*.

After the sculpting operations are performed, a topography (Figs 9.6 and 9.7) of the sculpted eye may be taken to show the difference curvature in zones of 6 mm and zone 4 mm. The doctor then examines the patient distance visual acuity and measures near visual acuity. If further errors are found, further sculpting is performed.

As shown, with this LASIK technique (PARM*) the corneal curvature is modified, creating a bilateral bifocal cornea. In order to have a high quality of vision, corneal keratometry should not be modified up to 48 D. Corneas with more than 48 D produce undesired optical alterations like glare, halos, decreased visual acuity and decreased contrast sensitivity. For each hypermetropic diopter corrected, the corneal curvature increases in 0.89 keratometric diopters as an average, that is why it is recommended to treat patients with keratometry in the range between 41 to 43 D to obtain postoperatively curves under 48 D. The corneal flap performed with the microkeratome must be between 8.5 to 9.5 mm in order to have an available corneal surface for treatment of at least 8 mm., this way the

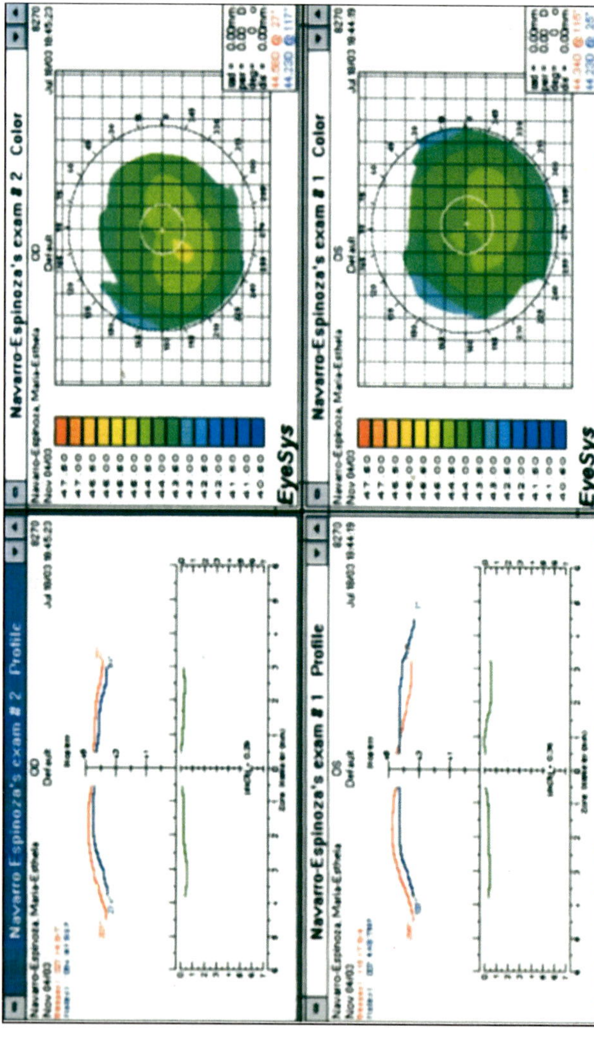

Fig. 9.6: Topography of patient treated with PARM* technique (Before treatment)

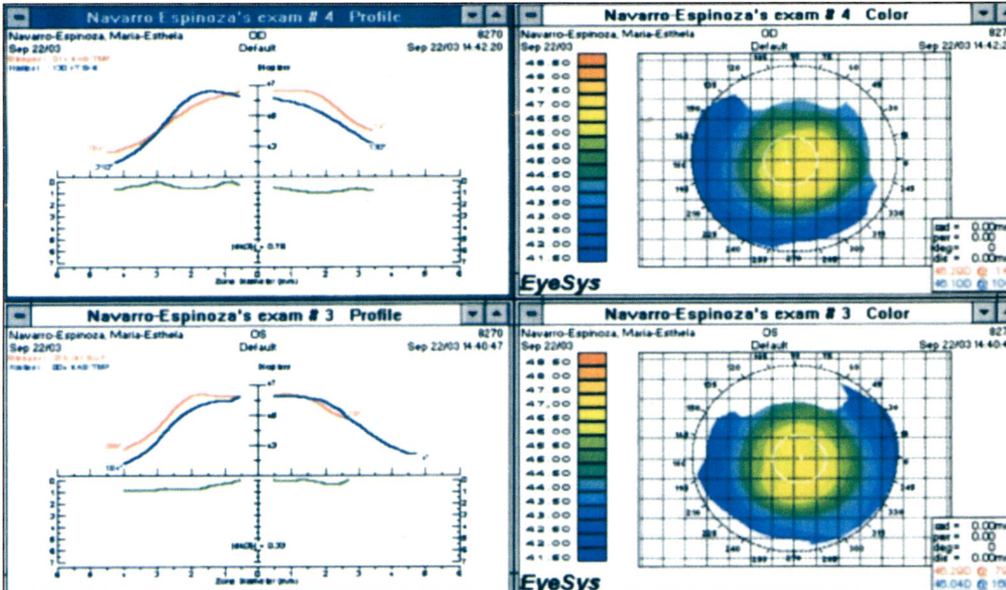

Fig. 9.7: Topography of patient treated with PARM* technique (After treatment)

laser beam does not touch the hinge of the flap. Pachymetry is not fundamental for this treatment, but it is the focusing ability of the eye as previously discussed.

PARM* has been used to treat patients with 20/20 distance vision and addition of +3.5 D; for hypermetropic patients up to +3.5 D in order to treat the addition for presbyopia, always taking into account the preoperatively keratometric measurement.

If astigmatism is present, it is recommended to use as a limit 2.50 D and in myopic patients the limit is –4.00 D. Because of the corneal shape produced after the surgery, there is an induced astigmatism between 0.50 to 0.75 D, which could decrease one or two lines of no corrected visual acuity. The usual LASIK re-treatment average for myopia, astigmatism and hyperopia is 7 percent, in cases treated for presbyopia it is increased up to 22 percent as seen in Avalos and Rozaki´s patients in the first two years of trial; after modifying the nomogram this re-treatment percentage should diminish under the range of 12 percent. This group has not seen complications from the surgery, beside those already reported for regular LASIK technique.

In conclusion, PARM* provides an effective, safe, inexpensive and efficient device which provides for eliminating difficulties encountered with prior devices, solves problems and obtains new results in the art.

PARM EVALUATION OF 52 EYES

Pre- and Post-Treatment using the VISX S4 Excimer Laser

Pre- and post-LASIK evaluation in 52 eyes in the following parameters:

- Sphere (D)
- Cylinder (D)
- UCVA - Distance
- UCVA - Reading
- Keratometry K1 and K2
- Addition
- Re-Treatment (Enhancements)

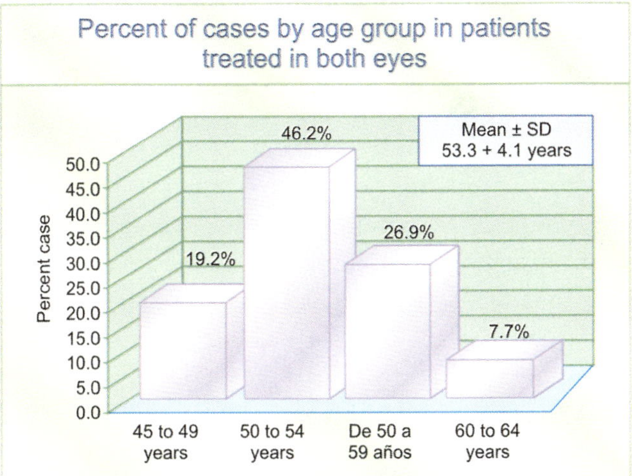

Fig. 9.8: Percent of cases by age group in patients treated in both eyes

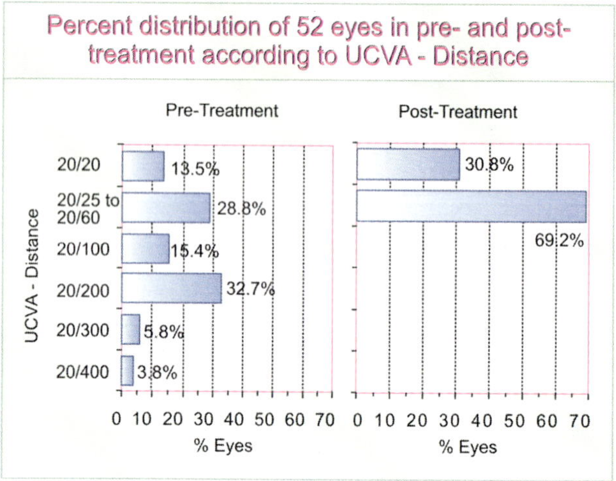

Fig. 9.9: Percent Distribution of 52 eyes in Pre- and Post-treatment according to UCVA - Distance

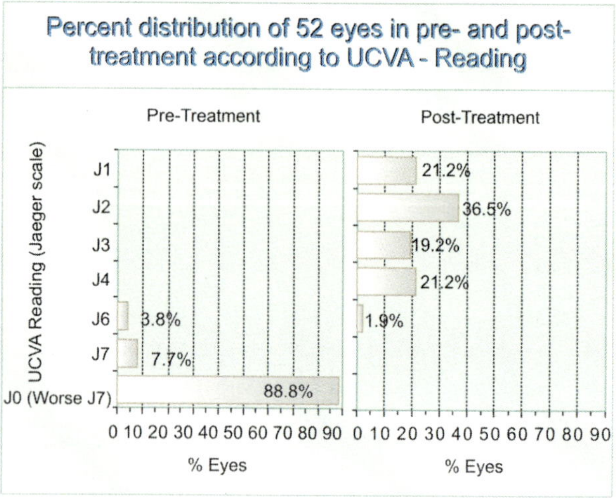

Fig. 9.10: Percent distribution of 52 eyes in pre- and post-treatment according to UCVA - Reading

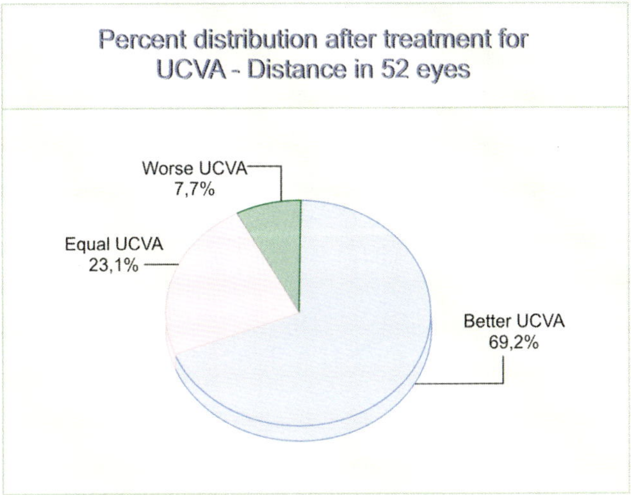

Fig. 9.11: Percent distribution after treatment for UCVA-Distance in 52 eyes

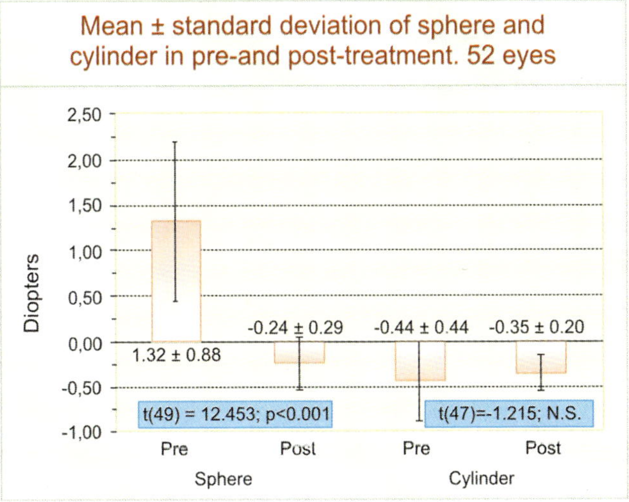

Fig. 9.12: Mean ± standard deviation of sphere and cylinder in pre- and post-treatment 52 eyes

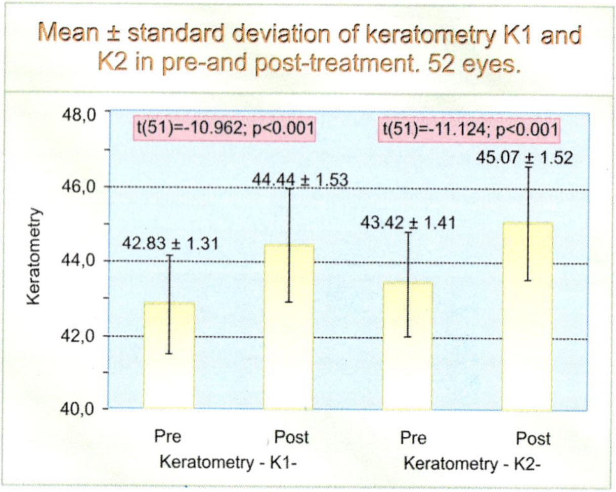

Fig. 9.13: Mean ± standard deviation of keratometry K1 and K2 in pre- and post-treatment 52 eyes

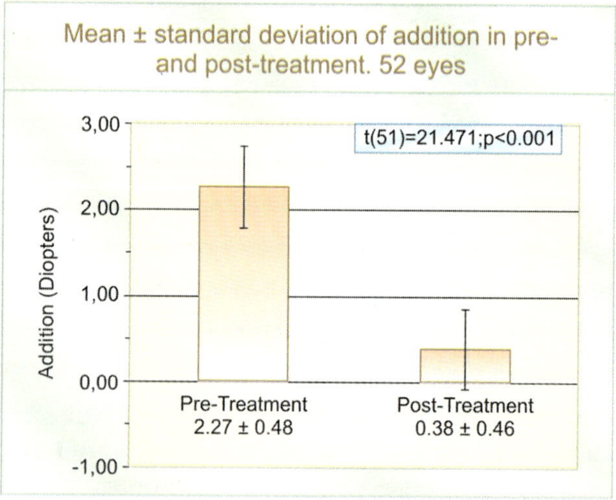

Fig. 9.14: Mean ± standard deviation of adition in pre- and post-treatment 52 eyes

Table 9.1: Initial and final results. Mean ± standard deviation (in units)

Statistical Evaluated parameter Significance	*Unit*	*Mean + standard deviation*		
		Initial	*Final*	
Sphere 0.001	Diopters	1.32 ± 0.88	–0.24 ± 0.29	p <
Cylinder	Diopters	–0.44 ± 0.44	–0.35 ± 0.20	NS
Keratometry K1	—	42.83 ± 1.31	44.44 ± 1.53	p <

Table 9.2: Comparative table (in percent) assuming initial value equal to 100%

		% Initial	*% Final*	*Change*
Sphere	%	100,0	–18,2	–118,2
Cylinder	%	100,0	79,5	–20,5
Keratometry K1	%	100,0	103,8	3,8
Keratometry K2	%	100,0	103,8	3,8
Addition	%	100,0	16,7	83,3

Statistical analysis consisted in the calculation of descriptive measures of central tendency and variability such as the mean and the standard deviation. In the case of ordinal variables, we calculated frequencies and percentages. Finally we made graphics to show the mean ± standard deviation, and frequency charts (Figs 9.8 to 9.14).

The parameters were compared between Pre- and Post-Treatment using Student's t-test for paired samples. Ordinal variables were compared using the chi-square test (Tables 9.1 and 9.2).

CHAPTER 10

Presbyopic LASIK for Myopia and Hyperopia "A New Optical Theory"—The Hypermultifocality of the Cornea

Frederic Hehn (France)

INTRODUCTION

Many techniques like: conductive keratoplastie, scleral incisions,[6] scleral expension band,[5] laser presbyopia reversal,[4] multifocal phakic IOL,[2] try to compensate presbyopia. Excimer laser is one of them.[3]

Cornea takes a great part of the accommodation process,[8] and then it doesn't astonish that some variations of the cornea shape can be used to compensate presbyopia.

Since many years, good results have been obtained in hyperopic eyes with excimer laser[1] for the both near and distant vision; in using central cornea for near vision and medium cornea for distant vision. But often this technique induce a little myopia and some discomfort for driving car due to the myosis in photopic conditions. This concept of distant vision in medium cornea and near vision in the center is not available in myopic eye. Then we tried to compensate presbyopia with the contrary concept: distant vision in central cornea and near vision in medium cornea like some authors do.[3]

Theoretical Basement

We propose a new optical theory: the hypermultifocality of cornea to explain our excellent results in presby-LASIK.

George O Waring[7] has described 4 anatomic zones of the cornea: central optical 0-4 mm OZ (optical zone), paracentral "medium" 4-8 mm OZ, peripheral 9-11 mm OZ and limbal 12 mm OZ. We have to describe 3 refractive optical zones.

In central cornea there is no spherical aberration. Infinity focus on macula without using lens accommodation. In central cornea, with the lens accommodation, the near vision is very precise because there is a lot of luminosity then also a good contrast sensitivity.

But is there another way to see a middle or near object without using lens accommodation? Yes there is, it's the "hyper-multifocality" of cornea due to the spherical aberration. It's well known that spherical aberrations are bad for distant vision because they give a big blur circle.

On the contrary, spherical aberration can be useful for middle vision. If you choice a P point of the medium cornea more than 4 mm OZ , of course there are spherical aberration, and the infinity do not focus on macula, but focus in front of the macula.

Due to the Fresnel-Descartes law **n1sin1 = n2sin2** we can find a "O" object which can focus on macula without lens accommodation. Many others object can focus on macula also without using lens accommodation.

That's I call "hyper-multifocality" of the medium cornea. Then at any time many object's planes focus together on macula without accommodation. The choice of the sharp image on the retina is a brain selection.

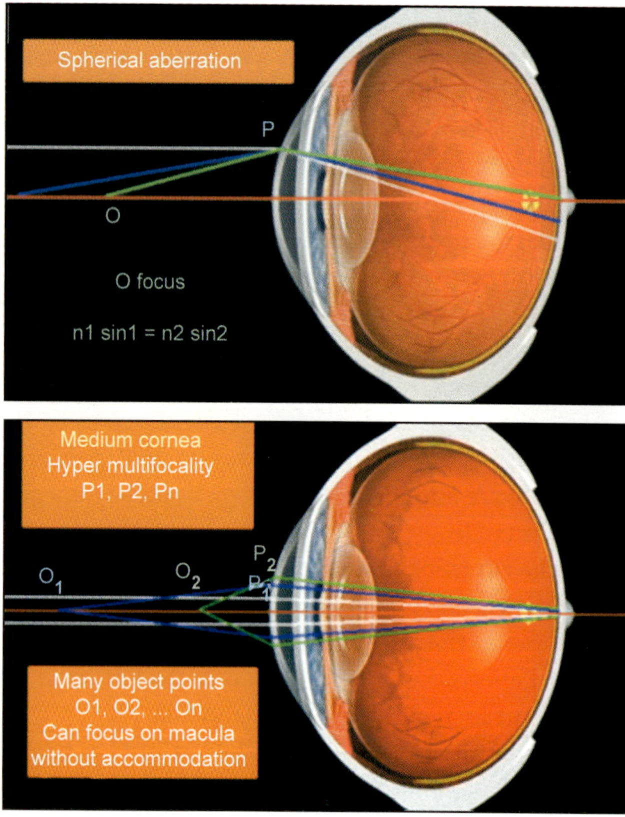

Fig. 10.1

The hyper-multifocality of the medium cornea expands the depth of focus. Evidently the nearest of the eye the object is, the more peripheral on the cornea is the focus point. Then it's a limited process, if the object is too near of the eye , the theoric focus point

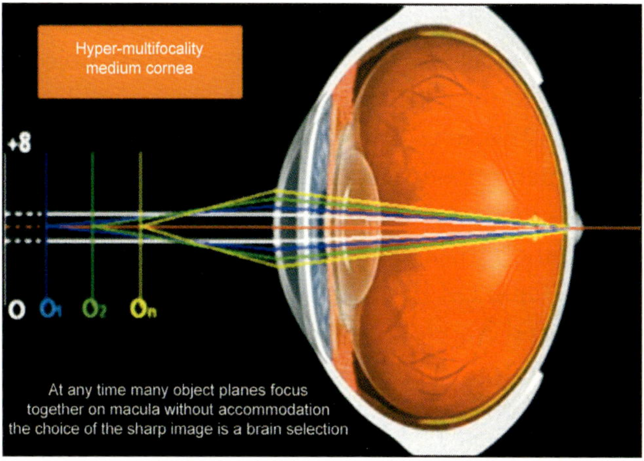

Fig. 10.2

will be too peripheral on the cornea and give no retinal image due to the pupil filter and the very low level of luminosity entrance inside the eye.

A proof? I can give you more than one. If you use a pin hole you lost depth of focus; it's very simple and every body can perform it.

A second proof is in concern with the pseudophakic emmetropic patient. Evidently it occurs in this case a very good distant vision, but also a good middle vision with a useful depth of focus, the only lack is the near vision. This good middle vision and depth of focus cannot be due to the central cornea and then consequently are due to the natural hyper-multifocality of the medium cornea.

Then I affirm: "In using spherical aberration it's possible to see a middle distant or a near object by medium cornea without using lens accommodation"

With this new concept, I had to find a constant keratometric zone, that's to say, a spherical cornea zone to use spherical aberration. We have analyzed 50 non-astigmatic cornea, and found a constant keratometry on a 6.0 mm OZ [min 5.00, max 7.00].

We find 3 optical zones for 3 refractive effects.

1. **Central [0 to 4]** for distant vision
2. **Medium [4 to 6]**
   spherical aberrations give hyper-multifocality for midle and near vision
3. **Peripheral [6 to 12]**
   there are spherical aberrations but the negative asphericity and pupil filter give no refractive effect. It's only useful for visual field, luminosity and contrast sensitivity.

PRESBY-LASIK TECHNIQUE

Our Presby-LASIK technique enhance natural property of hyper-multifocality of the medium cornea to focus on near objects without lens accommodation.

We are using now the high speed and precision wavelight allegretto Eye Q. The ablation profile is aspheric due to the wavefront optimized ablation profile. In central cornea a circular beam is being projected on the cornea but in medium and peripheral cornea the ellipse surface of the excimer laser treatment covers a larger area, resulting in a lower energy density. The lower ablation rate causes a spherical aberration resulting in poor night vision. The allegretto wave algorithm compensates for this.

The presby-LASIK first step is to steepen medium and central cornea for near and middle vision by a hyperopic 6.5 mm OZ treatment and 9.00 mm total treatment zone. The second step is to flatten central cornea for distant vision by a myopic 5.0 mm OZ treatment and 5.60 mm total treatment zone.

With this presby-LASIK technique, you can treat plus 3 diopters even at forty five years old to treat the present and the future presbyopia. Because the more you steepen the medium cornea, the more you can flatten the central cornea.

Presby-LASIK is only possible if the mesopic pupil size is less than 5 mm width. That's often the case in patients more than 50 years old.

We treat patients from 45 years old until 70 years old with the same technique.

RESULTS

We show only 2 clinical results. Case one, an hyperopic eye +1.00 of a 55-year-old female. After laser there is a very good point spread function.

The corneal topography before and after laser show a perfect centration.

Good results: 18/20 J2 monocular UCVA.

Case two, a 60 years old female, myopic –5.50 diopter. There is no increase in high order aberration after laser, but a gentle increase of second defocus (C12) C twelve = Z°4 " spherical aberration".

It remains also a C4 defocus – 3.25. It's only an aberrometric measurement but not a real value because the clinical refraction is plano. This measure is due to the steep curve of the medium cornea induced by the presby-LASIK treatment.

The corneal topography is perfectly centred and progressive with smooth transitions. The result is perfect, a very little point spread function. Patient has no glare and no halos. 20/20 J1 monocular UCVA.

DISCUSSION

In one hand, this kind of middle or near vision, in using the hyper-multifocality of the medium cornea, is tiredless because there is a passive view. But this view mode needs a lot of luminosity for a good contrast and depends on pupil size. In another hand the near vision in central cornea which use lens accommodation is tiredness because it's due to a muscular effort; but this kind of near vision is more precise because more luminosity can go inside the eye by central cornea than it can by medium cornea.

The results were good in the both myopic and hyperopic eye, because distant vision in central cornea and near vision in medium cornea seems to be more

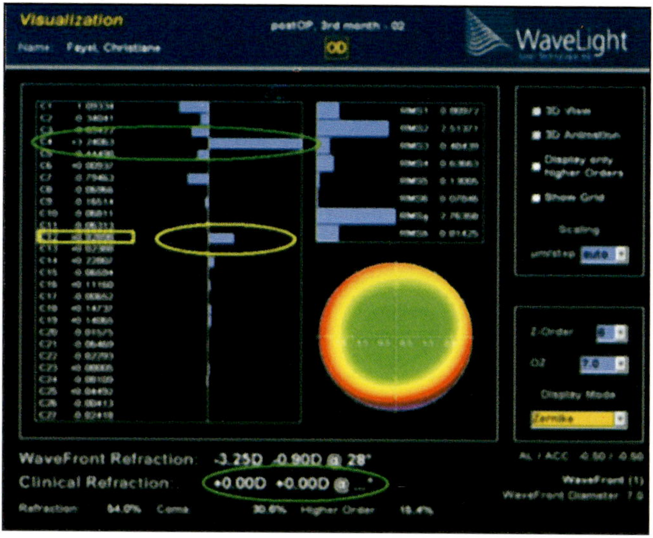

Fig. 10.3

efficient than the contrary concept, because it's use the natural property of hyper-multifocality of medium cornea to focus on middle and near vision, without using lens accommodation.

As the transitions zones are very, very progressives and smooth, patients get no glare and no halos. The pupil size has been controlled before laser treatment , and must be less than 5.00 mm width in mesopic condition. This technique give a good vision for distant vision whatever are the luminosity conditions.

The only restriction is the necessary of getting enough luminosity for a good contrast to near vision.

CONCLUSION

Our presby-LASIK technique build not a bifocal cornea but a continuous multifocal aspherical cornea that expand depth of focus to correct presbyopia. The next step is to treat pseudophakic eye with this presby-LASIK technique. Further studies must be done to confirm the hyper-multifocality theory and clinical results.

REFERENCES

1. Alió JL, Cimberle M. Presby-LASIK is an option for hyperopic presbyopic patients, surgeon says. Ocular surgery news, 30, November 2004.
2. Baikoff G, Matach G, Fontaine A, Ferraz C, Spera C. Correction of presbyopia with refractive multifocal phakic intraocular lenses. J Cataract Refract Surg 2004; 30: 1454-60.
3. Bruce Jackson W, Agarwal A, Avalos G. Multifocal LASIK offers multitude of options for treating presbyopia. Eurotimes, 31, October 2003.
4. Kadambi V, Lin JT. Clinical results of laser presbyopia reversal using the Optivision infrared laser in: Agarwal A, ed, Presbyopia; a Surgical Textbook. Thorofare, NJ, Slack, 2002; 133-35.
5. Mathiews S. Scleral expension surgery does not restore accommodation in human presbyopia. Ophthalmology 1999, 106; number 5, 873-77.
6. Schachar RA. Cause and treatment of presbyopia with a method for increasing amplitude of accommodation. Ann Ophthalmol 1992; 26:445-47, 452.
7. Waring III GO. Refractive keratotomy for myopia and astigmatism. Mosby – year book 1992, Chapter 3 page 49.
8. Yasuda A, Yamaguchi T, Ohkoshi K. Changes in corneal curvature in accommodation. J Cataract Refract Surg 2003;29:1297-1301.

CHAPTER 11

Conductive Keratoplasty for Presbyopia

Roberto Pinelli (Italy)

INTRODUCTION

Conductive keratoplasty (CK) with the ViewPoint System from Refractec, Inc. (Irvine, California) is a non-laser, radiofrequency-based procedure for treating presbyopia that avoids LASIK-associated complications, as well as many of the disadvantages of traditional monovision. High frequency (350 kHz) energy is delivered into the stroma with a specially designed contact probe. The temperature and duration of the radiofrequency energy applied by the probe is optimal for collagen shrinkage without necrosis.

Conductive keratoplasty requires no ablation or incisions, does not invade the central cornea, cause flap-related complications, compromise the integrity or structure of the cornea, or cause dry eye or central haze.

CK has been used primarily to treat low to moderate hyperopia[1-3] and to reduce the symptoms of presbyopia in presbyopic hyperopes (+1.00 to +2.25 D) or emmetropes through induction of mild myopia in the non-dominant eye.[4] Other potential uses of the CK technique under investigation include treatment of over- or undercorrections following LASIK or other excimer laser procedures, enhancing outcomes of cataract surgery, and treating astigmatism.

This chapter will briefly review the history of the CK procedure, explain how the system works and the surgical technique and procedures used by this author, and review the US clinical trial results for the treatment of presbyopia.

HISTORY

Thermokeratoplasty techniques aim to change corneal curvature through the application of heat, which shrinks corneal collagen. There were several attempts in the 1980s to use thermokeratoplasty to change corneal refraction in humans, but these were largely unsuccessful.[5-12]

Following the 1990 report by Seiler and associates of stable corneal steepening achieved in blind eyes with a pulsed holmium:YAG laser used in the contact mode,[13] Sunrise Technologies of Fremont, California, began to develop a non-contact method of holmium: YAG laser treatment for hyperopia. US clinical studies with two-year follow-up were published in 1996 and 1997[14-15] and the device was ultimately approved for use in the US in 2000, based on a study cohort of 612 eyes, with 80 percent available for analysis at 12 months and only 12 percent at 24 months postoperatively.[16]

Over time, LTK became unpopular because it lacked predictability and stability. The manufacturer went out of business and the Hyperion device is no longer manufactured.

Also in the 1990s, Antonio Mendez, MD, studied radiofrequency as an alternative to procedures that applied heat directly to the corneal surface.[17] His success in denaturing collagen and steepening the cornea led to the development of Refractec's ViewPoint CK System.

Unlike previous thermokeratoplasty methods that used a laser to generate heat intrastromally, conductive keratoplasty with the ViewPoint CK System uses radiofrequency energy to shrink corneal collagen.

A precise amount of radiofrequency energy is applied through a 450 × 90-μm contact probe inserted into the peripheral corneal stroma. Treatment is applied in a ring pattern outside of the visual axis at a defined number of treatment spots, with a greater number of spots applied to achieve a greater effect.

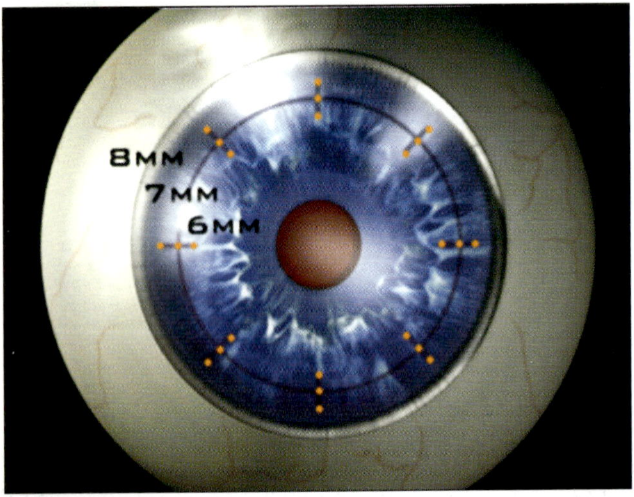

Fig. 11.1: Ring pattern outside the visual axis. This shows the optical zone marks made by the marker to guide the surgeon in placement of the treatment spots. A circular mark is made on the 7 mm optical zone with the CK marker. An inner hatch mark lies on the 6 mm and an outer hatch mark on the 8 mm optical zone

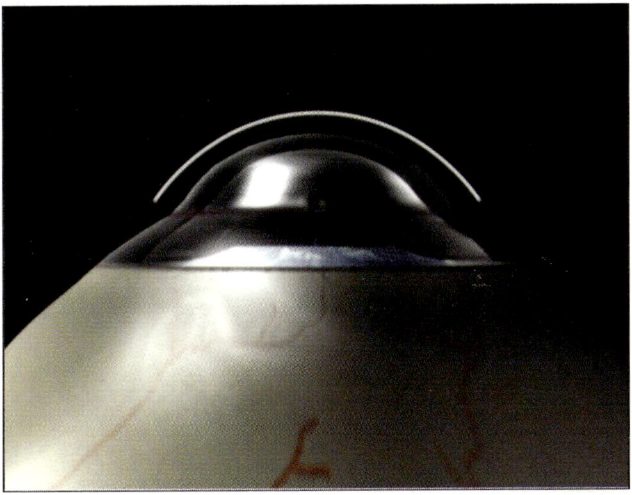

Fig. 11.2: The central cornea steepens. The conductive keratoplasty technique cinches the peripheral cornea which increases the curvature of the central cornea

A full circle of treatment spots acts like a belt tightening the cornea in the periphery so that the central cornea steepens.

During conductive keratoplasty treatment, corneal tissue is exposed to the same temperature at the bottom of the probe as at the corneal surface. The footprint after conductive keratoplasty is cylindrical and extends deep into the stroma to approximately 80 percent depth. This is in contrast to the conical stromal footprint made with the LTK technique.

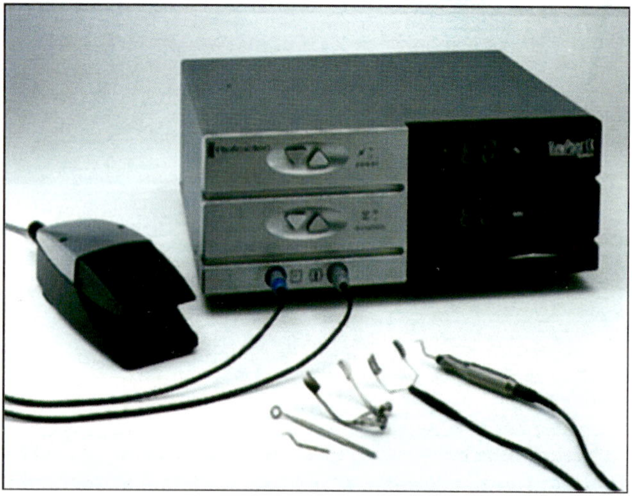

Fig. 11.3: The ViewPoint CK system. The ViewPoint™ CK system from Refractec, Inc. consists of a portable console, a corneal marker, choice of lid specula, a handpiece that holds the Keratoplast™ tip, and a foot pedal

THE CK SYSTEM

The ViewPoint CK System (Fig. 11.3) used to perform the CK procedure consists of a radiofrequency energy-generating console, a reusable, pen-shaped handpiece attached by a removable cable and connector, a foot pedal that controls the release of energy, a corneal marker, and a speculum that provides a large surface for an electrical return path.

Attached to the probe is a single-use, disposable, stainless steel, Keratoplast tip, 90 µm in diameter and 450 µm long, that delivers the current directly to the

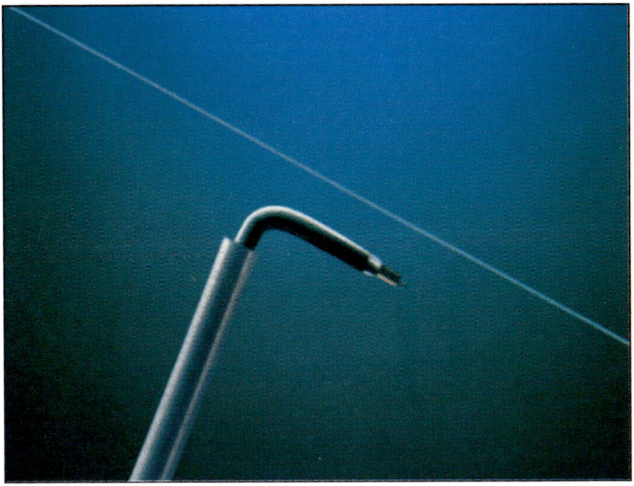

Fig. 11.4: The Keratoplast tip blue suture. The Keratoplast™ tip, (shown next to a 7-0 suture). The tip is 450 μm long and 90 μm wide and is used to deliver radiofrequency energy into the corneal stroma at the marked treatment points. A cuff on the probe assures correct depth of penetration

corneal stroma (Fig. 11.4). The tip has a proximal bend of 45° and a distal bend of 90° to allow access to the cornea over the patient's brow and nasal regions. At the very distal portion of the tip is an insulated stainless steel stop (cuff) that controls depth of penetration.

Treatment application of 0.6 seconds per spot causes the surrounding tissue to undergo a temperature increase. As the heated tissue dehydrates, its resistance to radiofrequency current increases. Since current seeks the path of least resistance, the current path moves up the shaft of the Keratoplast tip. Tissue heating progresses from bottom (approximately 80% of the depth

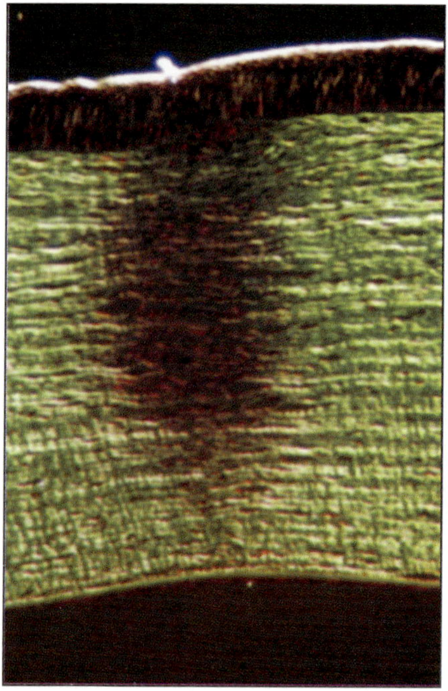

Fig. 11.5: Thermal lesion on the cornea. A polarized light micrograph of a histological section from a pig cornea, seven days after CK treatment. The footprint (dark region) is cylindrical and approximately 80 percent of corneal depth. Deep treatment penetration contributes to permanence of effect

of the stroma) to top (corneal surface), and creates a thermal lesion that is uniformly cylindrical (Fig. 11.5).

THE NEARVISION CK PROCEDURE

Conductive keratoplasty for presbyopic correction is often referred to as NearVision CK. For this procedure, patients should be 40 years old or older and presbyopic. Preoperative testing includes slit-lamp examination, keratometry, pachymetry, corneal topography, dominance assessment, near and distance vision assessment, and monovision tolerance assessment.

Vision should be correctable to 20/40 or better, and there should be no more than 0.75 D of refractive astigmatism, as determined by cycloplegic refraction. Contact lens wearers should have a stable refraction and should discontinue lens use for two (soft) to three (hard or gas permeable) weeks before the procedure. Evidence of monovision success from previous contact lens monovision, a contact lens trial, the loose-lens test, or other preoperative testing is an important factor in patient selection.

For near vision correction in presbyopic emmetropes and hyperopes, the goal is to overcorrect the nondominant eye by inducing slight to moderate myopia, –1.0 to –2.0 D (myopic endpoint) through the application of 8 to 24 CK treatment spots. If the dominant eye is significantly hyperopic, it can be targeted for a distance correction of +0.50 to –0.25 D. Treated patients display a reduction of symptoms of presbyopia without compromising binocular functional distance vision.

At the Institute, we begin on the day of surgery by verifying that the patient's pachymetry measurement is at least 560 µm at the 6 mm optical zone. After checking the device settings, the Keratoplast tip is interested into the handpiece and inspected under a microscope. I use foamed alcohol on my hands before performing CK; I do not use gloves for this procedure.

Preoperatively, we administer one drop of Tobradex followed by one drop of topical anesthetic (proparacaine) three times at five minute intervals. A lid speculum is placed in the eye to obtain maximal exposure and provide the electrical return path. To ensure direct contact of the speculum with the lids, we do not drape.

With the patient fixating under the excimer laser microscope, the surgeon should center carefully on the pupil and mark the eye. Proper centration is critical to avoiding the induction of astigmatism. We use gentian violet ink and the standard CK marker, although there is also a newer 24-point marker developed by Dr Strauss. The marker should be applied straight down and then lifted straight up after a short pause to obtain clear marking. After marking, the surgeon dries the corneal surface and then uses a dry fiber-free sponge to remove any excess ink.

The surgeon then inserts the Keratoplast tip into the stroma at defined spots in a ring pattern around the peripheral cornea. At the Institute, we use the nomogram and sequence shown in Figure 11.6. The handpiece should be held in the dominant hand in a relaxed position, with the index finger of the opposite hand used to steady it, if necessary. At the marked treatment spot, tip the body of the handpiece approximately tangential to the optical zone mark. The Keratoplast

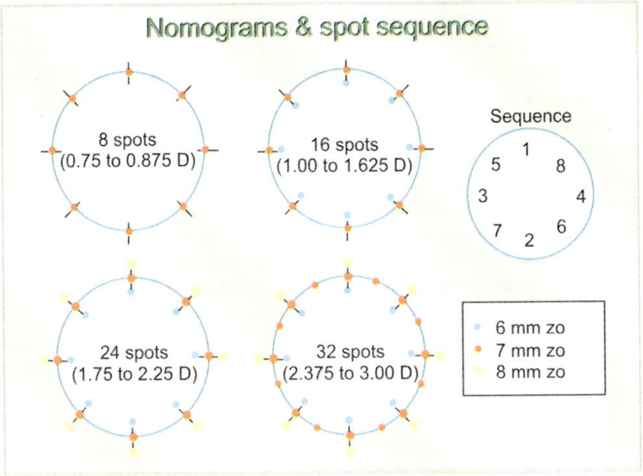

Fig. 11.6: Nomograms and spot sequence used at the istituto Laser Microchirurgia Oculare – Brescia - Italy. According to the nomogram in use at the ILMO, most patients need 8-16 spots for presbyopic correction

tip should be perpendicular to the corneal surface to ensure full depth of penetration. The cuff around the probe, which settles perpendicular to the cornea, helps to achieve perpendicular placement.

We apply uniform downward pressure until the tip penetrates the stroma. Then, energy is applied by depressing the foot pedal. During treatment, the amount of pressure applied is very important. Recent studies have shown that a light touch or neutral pressure technique, in which the cornea is indented and the ring light displaced as little as possible, is ideal for most primary treatments.

Spots should be applied smoothly and evenly. Begin treatment at the 12 o'clock position and continue, following the sequence in Figure 11.6, until the full ring of spots has been completed for that optical zone. Each spot should be applied parallel to the others in that ring and to those in the other optical zones. When applying a second or third ring of treatment, aim for precise radial alignment of treatment spots so that the spots in each ring just barely touch each other. Any tissue debris that accumulates on the tip can be removed with a fiber-free sponge.

If the ring light indicates that any cylinder has been induced during the procedure, a balancing spot can be placed intraoperatively. In total, the CK procedure takes only a few minutes to complete.

Postoperatively, we follow the same regimen that we use for LASIK: One drop of Tobradex four times daily for one week and artificial tears as needed for one month. At the first follow-up visit (Day 1), patients may experience mild foreign body sensation, possibly with photophobia. This usually resolves in 24 to 48 hours. There may also be some edema, which may persist through the next follow-up visit, at one to two weeks postoperative. At this point, the patient's visual acuity is generally good, although there will be further improvement. The patient may need reassurance that it will continue to get better. If there is any late-developing astigmatism, a balancing spot can be added. By the four to six week follow-up visit, patients should have no discomfort or edema, and good near and distance visual acuity. In fact, vision is often better than would be expected with the measured refraction. Enhancement can be discussed at this visit, if necessary.

CLINICAL RESULTS

The FDA clinical study for approval of NearVision CK for the correction of presbyopia was conducted at five sites in the United States. A total of 150 presbyopic patients (188 eyes) were enrolled and treated with CK. One hundred twelve patients were treated unilaterally for near vision correction; 38 patients were treated bilaterally for distance correction in one eye and near in the other. The average age was 53 years old; 96 percent of all patients were Caucasian, and 61 percent were female. The mean intended correction for eyes treated for near was +2.03 D ± 0.63 D (range +0.75 D to 3.00 D).

Visual Acuity

Of the eyes treated for near, 81 percent had J2 or better binocular UCVA-Near at six months; 77 percent at 12 months. For UCVA-Near of J3 or better, the percentage was 90 percent and 89 percent, compared with only (15%) that had this uncorrected binocular near acuity preoperatively (Fig. 11.7).

Binocular UCVA-Distance results showed 95 percent and 97 percent with 20/20 or better acuity at 6 and 12 months, respectively, 100 percent and 98 percent

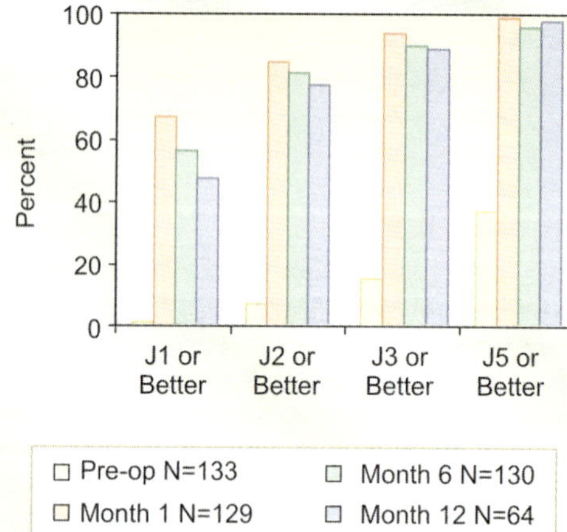

Fig. 11.7: Binocular UCVA-Near CK US FDA Presbyopia Study. Treatment range (1.00 to 2.25 D). Binocular UCVA-Near following CK presbyopia treatment

with 20/25 or better, and 100 percent with 20/32 or better (Fig. 11.8).

The combination of binocular UCVA-Distance of 20/20 or better with UCVA-Near of J2 or better was achieved by 100 of 130 eyes (77%) at six months and 48 of 64 eyes (75%) at 12 months. Approximately 90 percent of patients could see binocularly 20/20 or better distance and J3 or better near uncorrected (Fig. 11.9).

Safety

At one month, 2 percent of the treated eyes showed a loss of more than two lines of BSCVA-Distance; this incidence fell to zero percent for all subsequent months.

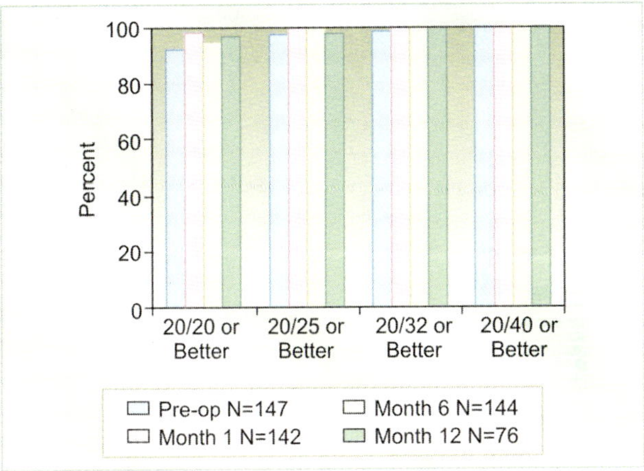

Fig. 11.8: Binocular UCVA-Distance CK US FDA Presbyopia Study. All subjects treated for near with Tx range 1.00 to 2.25 D. Binocular UCVA-Distance following CK presbyopia treatment

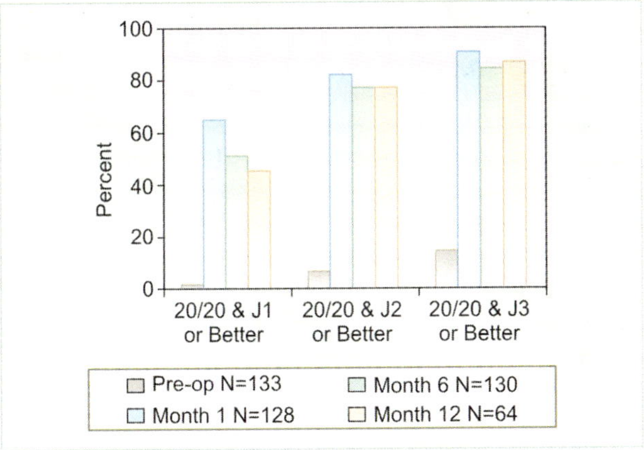

Fig. 11.9: Binocular UCVA 20/20 Distance and Near CK US FDA Presbyopia Study. All subjects treated for near treatment range +1.00 to +2.25 D. Binocular Combined UCVA-Distance and Near following CK presbyopia treatment

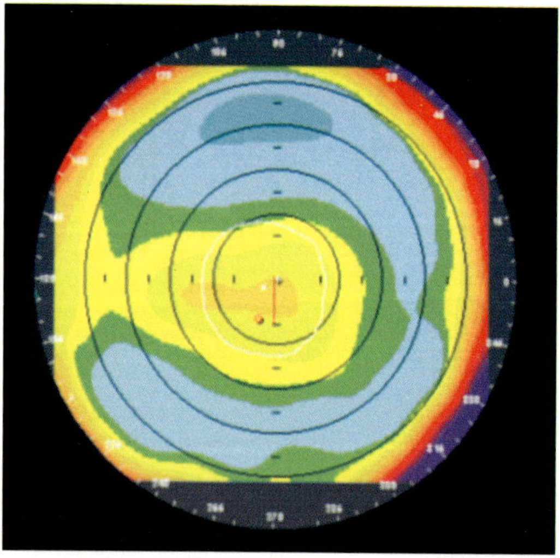

Fig. 11.10: Preoperative topography

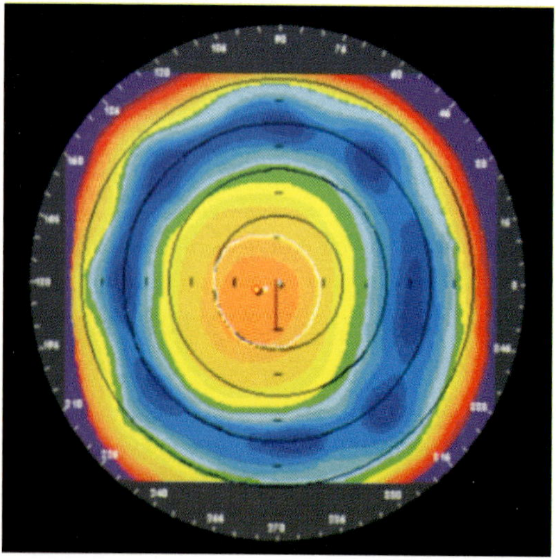

Fig. 11.11: One year postoperative topography

There were no cases of BSCVA worse than 20/40, increases of $\geq$ 2.00 D of cylinder, or eyes that had 20/20 or better BSCVA preoperatively that had worse than 20/25 postoperatively. Postoperative increases in absolute cylinder were generally 1.50 D or less and decreased with time. No intraoperative complications or adverse events occurred during any of the surgeries.

Vision Quality and Patient Satisfaction

Of the patients who had eyes treated for near, 97 percent reported improvement in quality of vision at one month; 98 percent at 12 months. At these time periods, a total of 85 percent and 84 percent reported being satisfied or very satisfied with their outcome. All patients reported fair to excellent quality of depth perception. Mesopic contrast sensitivity testing with and without glare showed that contrast sensitivity was maintained following CK.

A patient questionnaire about spectacle use following the CK procedure showed that most patients had significantly reduced their dependence on spectacles for common daily tasks. After the CK procedure, 90 percent of patients could use a computer without spectacles, 86 percent could read menus, and 86 percent could read newspaper-sized print (approximately J5 or 8-point font size). This reinforces the goal of the CK procedure, to allow the patient to perform most daily tasks without spectacles.

SUMMARY

Conductive keratoplasty is a non-laser procedure for changing corneal curvature to treat presbyopia, low to moderate spherical hyperopia, and other refractive conditions. The largest potential population for CK appears to be the presbyopes, many of whom are interested in a non-laser procedure that can extend the period of spectacle-free near vision.

The US FDA multicenter study showed that CK was safe and effective for improving near vision in presbyopic patients, and the clinical results at our Institute have been similarly excellent.

Importantly, none of the disadvantages typically associated with monovision seem to occur with NearVision CK. Depth perception is maintained, binocular corrected distance acuity is generally better than preoperative levels, and there is no loss of contrast sensitivity (quality of vision) from preoperative levels. Patient satisfaction is very high, and the vast majority of patients have binocular visual acuity of 20/20 or better at distance and J3 or better at near, for good functional vision without glasses.

NearVision CK is a safe, effective, and well-established approach to treating presbyopia and/or hyperopia. It also has the potential for treating other conditions. At the Institute, for example, we are treating keratoconus and astigmatism in post-cataract surgery patients by placing treatment spots on specifically chosen locations on the cornea. However, the surgeon must be highly experienced with conventional CK procedures before undertaking such procedures.

REFERENCES

1. McDonald MB, Davidorf J, Maloney RK, Manche EE, Hersh P. Conductive keratoplasty for the correction of low to moderate hyperopia: 1-year results on the first 54 eyes. Ophthalmology 2002;109:637-49.
2. McDonald MB, Hersh PS, Manche EE, Maloney RK, Davidorf J, Sabry M. Conductive keratoplasty for the correction of low to moderate hyperopia: US clinical trial 1-year results on 355 eyes. Ophthalmology 2002; 109:1978-89.
3. Asbell PA, Maloney RK, Davidorf J, Hersh P, McDonald M, Manche E. Conductive Keratoplasty Study Group. Conductive keratoplasty for the correction of hyperopia. Trans Am Ophthalmol Soc 2001;99:79-84.
4. McDonald MB, Durrie DS, Asbell PA, Maloney R, Nichamin L. Treatment of presbyopia with conductive keratoplasty: Six-month results of the 1-year United States FDA clinical trial. Cornea 2004;23:661-68.
5. Caster AI. The Fyodorov technique of hyperopia correction by thermal coagulation: A preliminary report. J Refract Surg 1988;4:105-08.
6. Neumann A, Sanders D, Salz J. Radial thermokeratoplasty for hyperopia. J Refract Corneal Surg 1989;5:50-54.
7. Neumann A, Fyodorov S, Sanders D. Radial thermokeratoplasty for the correction of hyperopia. J Refract Corneal Surg 1990;6:404-12.
8. Neumann A, Sanders D, Raanan M, DeLuca M. Hyperopic thermokeratoplasty: Clinical evaluation. J Cataract Refract Surg 1991;17:830-38.
9. Feldman S, Ellis W, Frucht-Pery J, et al. Regression of effect following radial thermokeratoplasty in humans. J Refract Surg 1995;18:288-91.

10. Rowsey JJ, Doss JD. Preliminary report of Los Alamos keratoplasty techniques. Ophthalmology 1981;88:755-60.
11. Rowsey JJ, Gaylor JR, Dahlstrom R, et al. Contact Intraocul Lens Med J 1980;6:1-12.
12. Rowsey JJ. Electrosurgical keratoplasty: Update and retraction. Invest Ophthalmol Vis Sci 1987;28 (suppl):224.
13. Seiler T, Matallana M, Bende T. Laser thermokeratoplasty by means of a pulsed holmium:YAG laser for hyperopic correction. Refract Corneal Surg 1990;6:355-59.
14. Koch DD, Abarca A, Villareal R, et al. Hyperopia correction by non-contact holmium:YAG laser thermokeratoplasty; clinical study with two year follow-up.
15. Koch D, Kohnen T, McDonnell P, et al. Hyperopia correction by noncontact holmium:YAG laser thermal keratoplasty. US Phase IIA Clinical Study with 2-year follow-up. Ophthalmology 1997;104:1938-47.
16. United States FDA PMA P990078. Hyperion LTK System Device Labeling, Sunrise Technologies, Fremont, California, May 2000.
17. Mendez A, Mendez Noble A. Conductive keratoplasty for the correction of hyperopia. In: Sher N (Ed). Surgery for Hyperopia and Presbyopia. Philadelphia: Williams and Wilkins: 1997;163-71.

CHAPTER 12

Aberrometric Corrections of Presbyopia

Franco Bartoli (Italy)

PRESBYOPIA AND ACCOMMODATION

The word presbyopia (which comes from Greek πρεσβυς οψ = old eye), identifies the age-related reduced ability in near vision.

In spite of last century's technical progress, the mechanisms of accommodation and the reason for which its decrease causes presbyopia remain a partly solved problem. Recently measurements with two different units (VISANTE OCT and UBM) confirm probably the Helmholtz's theory (Marchini).

There are two opposite theories:

1. *Helmholtz's theory (1855)* and subsequent modifications derive the accommodation from a decrease in zonular tension, with a relative curving of the crystalline lens front surface (greater refractive power) and an increase in its front-rear diameter. Presbyopia is due to a crystalline lens sclerosis (lack of elasticity) and to an atrophy of ciliar muscle with consequent impossibility to obtain such a curving (Fig. 12.1).
2. *Schachar's theory (1994)* assumes that zonula fibers can be divided into three groups: front, equatorial and rear fibers. Accommodation only involves the equatorial ones, while front and rear fibers have almost solely a support function. During the accommodation process there would be an increase in equatorial fibers tension and a decrease in that of front and rear ones; therefore, there is an increase in central curvature and a decrease in the peripheral

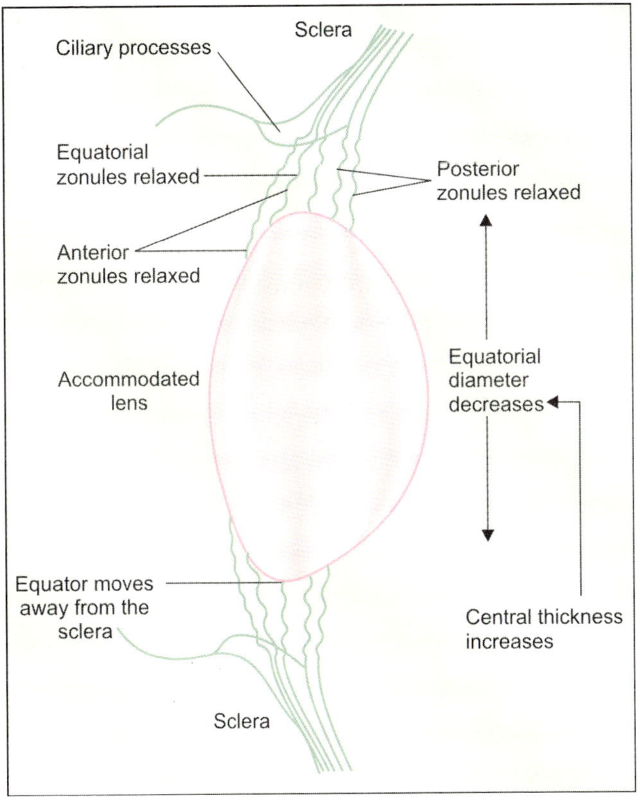

Fig. 12.1

one, related to an increase in front-rear diameter (thickness) of crystalline lens (Fig. 12.2). The loss of accommodation is bounded to the increase of crystalline lens equatorial volume (about 20 µm, per year) and to the consequent decrease in distance between the ciliary muscle body and the crystalline

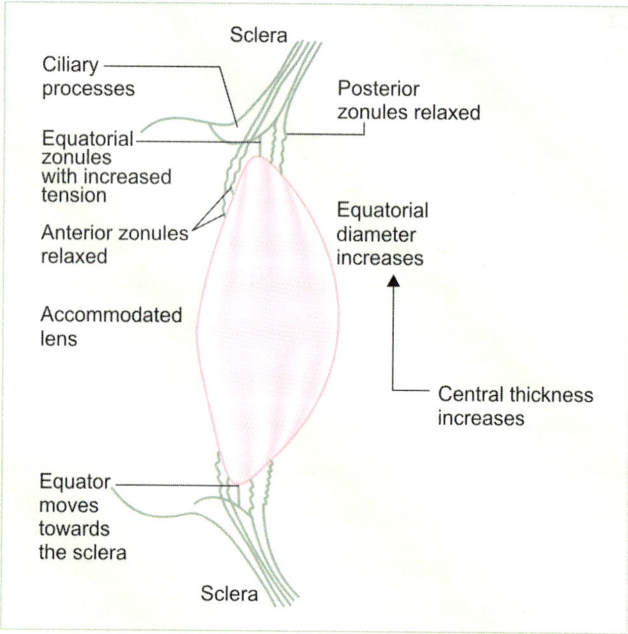

Fig. 12.2

lens equator, with relative loss of efficiency of tractional activity by the equatorial fibers.

According to the above theories, during the accommodation process the increased crystalline lens refractive power (accommodation) is caused by the increased curvature of the entire front surface (Helmholtz) or by an increase of the central one with a decrease in the peripheral one (Schachar). Theories apart, presbyopia correction has always been realized with positive lenses (either monofocal, bifocal, or multifocal) which guaranteed focus at about 30-40 cm.

After finding solutions for myopia, hypermetropy and astigmatism, in the last few years refractive surgery has been fighting for a new goal: Correct presbyopia. Schachar's hypothesis, based on practical experimentation (SEB), has started a race between all people involved in refractive surgery (manufacturers, ophthalmologists, etc.) towards a possible practical solution. Scleral expansion bands (Schachar) have been proposed to move the ciliary muscle away from the crystalline lens equator.

Excimer laser ablation assumes that the cornea, interpreted a glass lens, is transformed into a bifocal or multifocal lens. Another possible solution is monovision, and so on. For the last three years Bartoli have been proposing a slight different solution with excimer laser. Taking advantage of the newest aberrometric acquisitions, it offers a possible solution in this field.

SPHERICAL ABERRATION

When an optical system has an axis of revolution, the light rays emitted from a point P remain on the plane of incidence containing the axis and hit it again at a point P_1 (Fig. 12.3).

If the rays converge at 1, the plane of the pupil of entrance, which is perpendicular to the axis at C, the length C-I is defined as the height of incidence h. All

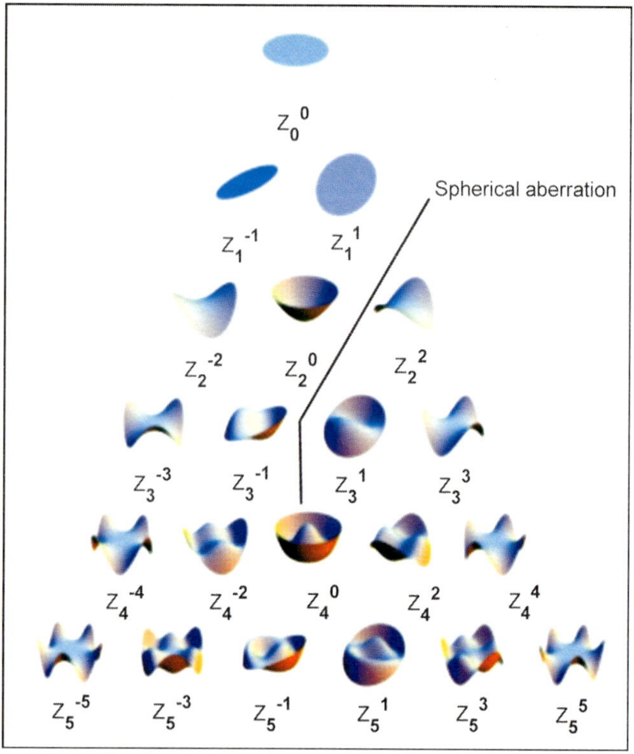

Fig. 12.3: Spherical aberration

rays of equal *h* that arrive from *P* reach a certain point P_1 (Fig. 12.4), but the position of this point is a function of *h*.

$$X^1 = a_o + a_1h + a_2h_2 + \dots \dots = a_o + \delta x^1$$

The coefficients *a* are functions of the abscissa *x*, the sources and the wavelength λ.

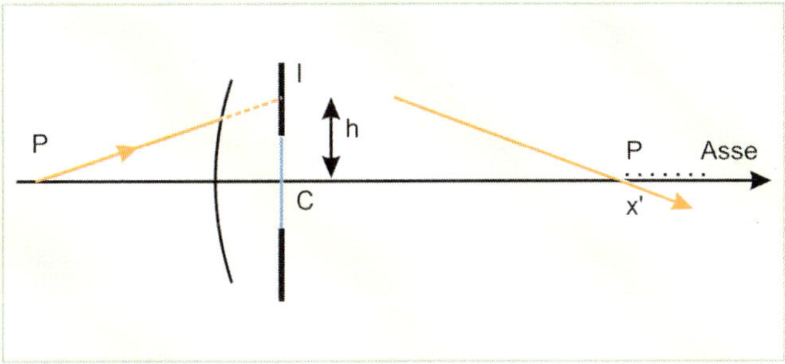

Fig. 12.4: Spherical aberration

The term a_o is the abscissa of the paraxial image or image according to Gauss's approximation, and corresponds to the value x^1 when h is infinitely small.

In the above formulation, the quantity δx^1, which unites all terms other than a_o, is called spherical aberration and expresses the divergence between the paraxial image and the point where the rays actually focus on the axis; it is a function of h, x and λ.

An optical system is called "correct" when spherical aberration is zero for a certain value of x and λ; this system is called stigmatic for the point object and the set λ. In most cases, the spherical diopter is not a correct system.

Spherical aberration is due to the fact that the peripheral regions of a lens have a refractive power different from that of the central areas. For example, in a biconvex lens the rays that hit a central area are focused at a greater distance and those that hit the peripheral area focus at a shorter distance from the lens (Fig. 12.5).

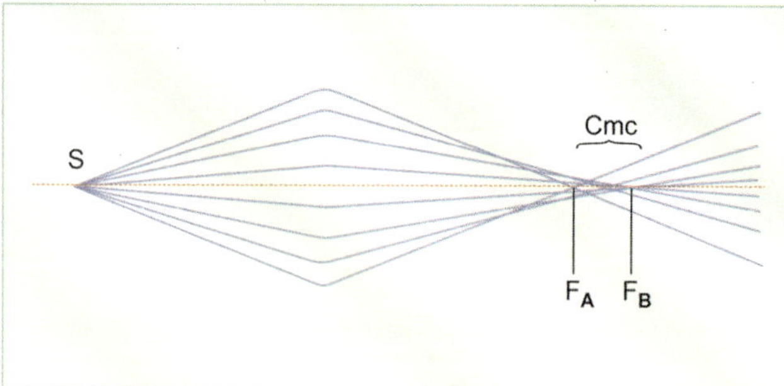

Fig. 12.5: Spherical aberration

There are two focus, one for the central rays and another for the peripheral rays. The distance between the two focus determines a triangular area called the caustic (Figs. 12.6 and 12.7).

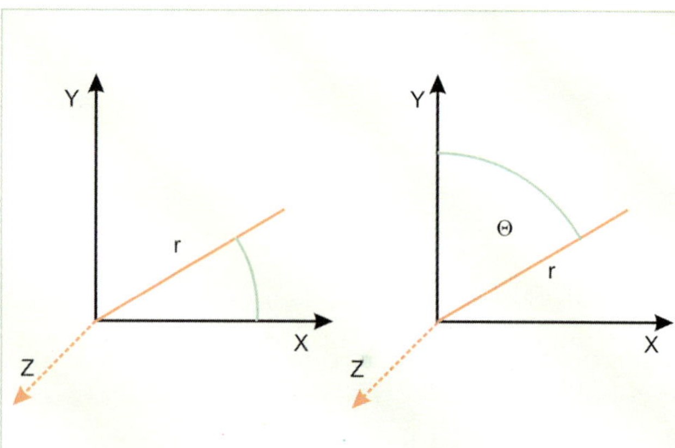

Fig. 12.6: OSA and Malacara.

OSA—coordinate system: $\sqrt{5}(6R^4 - 6R^2 + 1)$

WASCA (V1.26)—coordinate system: $6R^4 - 6R^2 + 1$

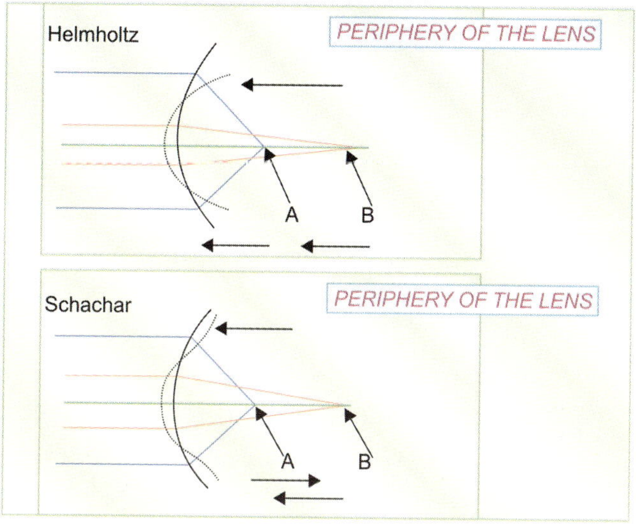

Fig. 12.7

In an incorrect system, the spherical aberration ($\delta\ x^1$) can be positive or negative. As h increases, P^1 moves towards or away from the light source, and the system is called overcorrect or undercorrect. The caustic defined as the surface fashioned from an outer envelope of light rays has its point P^1 in either one sense or the other, depending on whether there is overcorrection (Figs 12.8 and 12.9) or undercorrection (Figs 12.10 and 12.11).

In the last few years, depending on the calculation systems (WASCA or OSA) and thus on the aberrometer, front wave being equal, the same spherical aberration could be defined as positive or negative and even change its numeric value, inducing confusion. That is

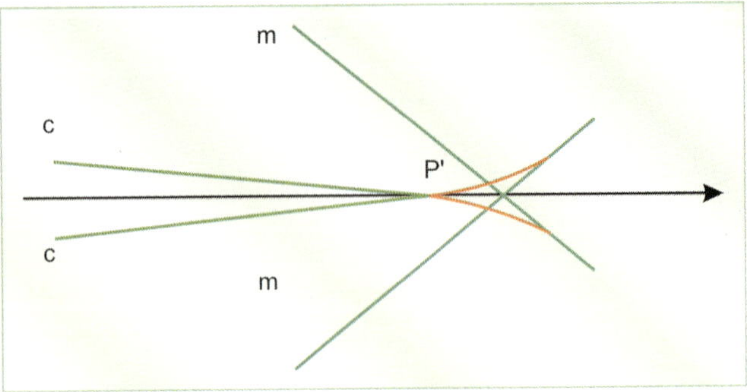

Fig. 12.8: Positive spherical aberration

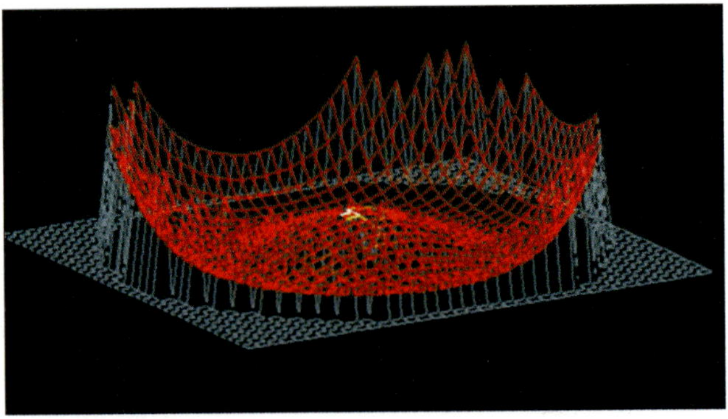

Fig. 12.9: 3-D image of positive spherical aberration

the reason why a conversion system has been prepared. It is always necessary to specify which one notation is used.

In our description results we always use the MALACARA notation :

1. When marginal rays focus is closer to the crystalline lens than paraxial rays, a positive spherical aberration is present.

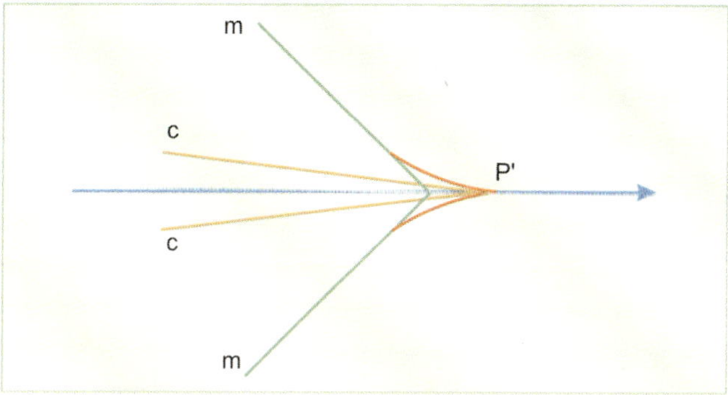

Fig. 12.10: Negative spherical aberration

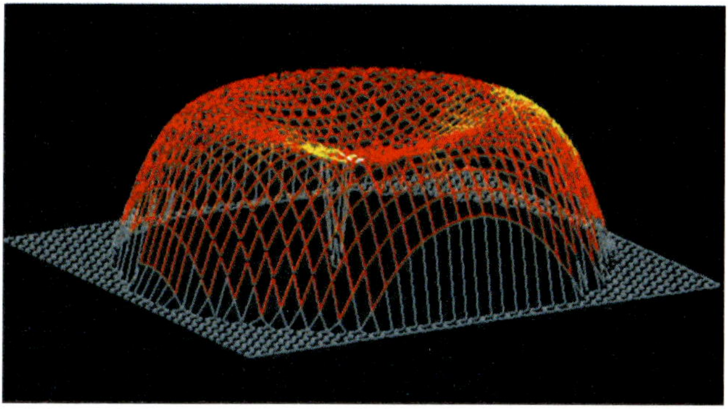

Fig. 12.11: 3D image of negative spherical aberration

2. When marginal rays focus is farther form the crystalline lens than that of paraxial rays, a negative spherical aberration is present.

Out of Helmholtz's and Schachar's theory, during accommodation, there is always positive spherical aberration induction, with two focus A and B identifying a caustic defined as the surface fashioned from an outer envelope of light rays.

Since the cornea of the eye is aspherical (correct optical system), spherical aberration is due to the lens. In accommodation at rest, spherical aberration is almost zero or slightly negative; during accommodation it increases and becomes positive. Hence, the eye's optical system is undercorrect in accommodation at rest and overcorrect during accommodation.

The Eye and the Spherical Aberration

In a study of the human eye in 1500 patients conducted with a WASCA aberrometer, spherical aberration was found to be zero or slightly negative in accommodation at rest (Pallicaris).

The cornea is a practically aspherical lens, as is the lens in the absence of accommodation. During accommodation, both for near vision or compensation of a hypermetropic defect for far vision, the central anterior surface of the lens curves, inducing positive spherical aberration.

With dynamic wavefront analysis using a WASCA aberrometer it was possible to quantify both accommodation (Fig. 12.12A) and induced positive spherical aberration (Figs 12.12B and 12.13); or impossibility of accommodation and apherical aberration induction in presbiopic eye (Fig. 12.14).

At this point, a direct correlation can be assumed between spherical aberration and accommodation. In confirmation of what was stated above, it can be shown that in presbyopes over 60 years of age there is no

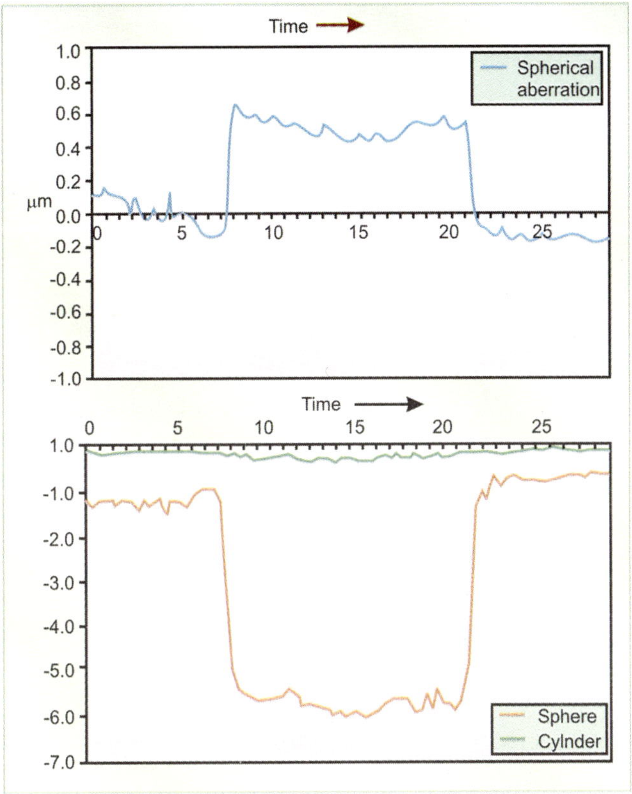

Figs 12.12A and B: Variation of spherical aberration during accommodation

increase in spherical aberration since they try to accommodate. Briefly:

1. In presbyopia there is a lack of accommodation with increasing age;

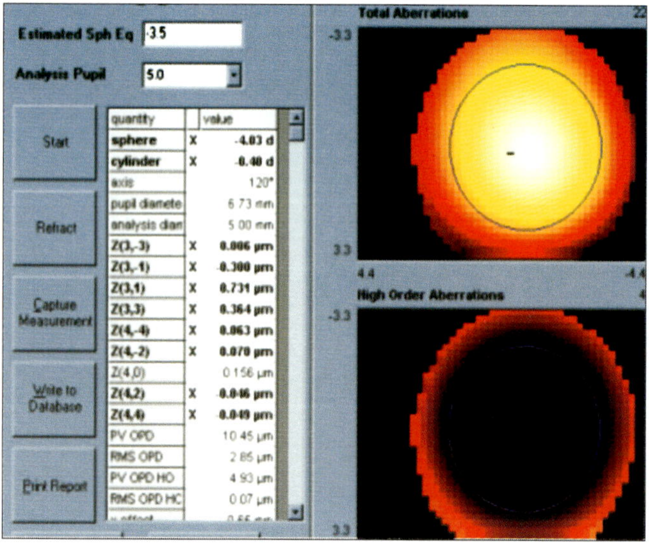

Fig. 12.13: Positive spherical aberration during accommodation (–4.03 Δ)

2. During accommodation there is a shift in spherical aberration from zero or negative to positive or only positivation of spherical aberration;
3. A close correlation exists between accommodation and spherical aberration;
4. In presbyopes, the loss of accommodation is accompanied by a loss of the ability to induce spherical aberration;
5. Inducing an increase in positive spherical aberration can compensate for the loss of accommodation in the presbyope.

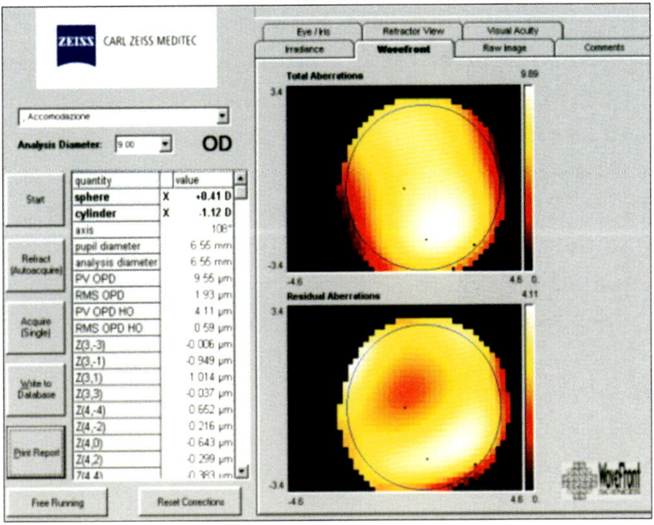

Fig. 12.14: In presbyop there is not accommodation and spherical aberration induction

To confirm what previously stated, the following experiment can be performed, on the basis that placing in front of the eye a neutral lens, the optical system is not modified (Peyman).

- Using an excimer laser, spherical aberration is induced on a neutral lens
- The lens is applied on a emmetrope, presbyopic patient
- The patient will have a normal distance vision and will acquire a good near vision.

Dynamic wavefront analysis allows accommodation to be objectively assessed and changes in the wavefront it induces, i.e. there is an increase of spherical aberration from almost zero or slightly negative to positive. In moderately hypermetropic patients in non-presbyopic age with good farsightedness and near-sightedness without corrective lenses, the correlation between the change of accommodation and the change of spherical aberration is particularly significant.

A young, moderately hypermetropic eye focuses far and near objects thanks to the increased curvature of the central anterior surface of the lens, with a relative induction of positive spherical aberration. The eye of the young hypermetrope is always in accommodation; it always has positive spherical aberration and a good quality of vision. It is evident that: **spherical aberration is the key**.

Wavefront analysis after hypermetropic photorefractive correction shows an increase and positivation of spherical aberration; conversely, after myopic correction it increases but still remains negative.

In hypermetropic presbyopes, circular corona refractive treatment corrects the refractive defect for far vision and also partially corrects the defect for near vision. If associated with aberrometric treatment, which corrects spherical aberration and raises it from negative to zero, a further increase is obtained with positivation of spherical aberration, thus fully correcting near vision. In addition, coma aberration is improved, with a subsequent enhancement of quality of vision. Hence, there is an evident correlation between hypermetropic treatment, positive spherical aberration and accommodation.

In the optical system of the eye, the first diopter (cornea) remains aspherical, the second (lens) does not; despite the induction of spherical aberration, the quality of the image does not deteriorate but improves instead, nor is there any alteration in contrast perception. The objective, therefore, is to make the presbyopic eye resemble a hypermetropic eye in constant accommodation by inducing a certain amount of spherical aberration on the cornea.

Research on spherical aberration and its measurement in the human eye has always been hampered by the fact that the optical system could only be studied from one side, unlike the examination of telescopic lenses or a photographic objective.

The first observations on spherical aberration in the human eye were made by Juren (1738) and the first measurements by Young (1801), and later studies by Tscherning and Gullstrand. But it was not until 1950 that an effective method was found to objectify measurements, wherein the image of a light source was formed on the retina and then used as a source of light to study aberrations of the eye as done with any objective. It was discovered that the light diffused by the retina suppresses the distribution of optical phase caused by the first passage of light through the eye, so that the results were referable only to the reverse/return trajectory.

During the early 1950s, Francon and Ivanoff (1951-1953) demonstrated that, contrary to previous thought, an increase of spherical aberration did not deteriorate the quality of the image. In fact, except for a small central area, the emerging wave was in concordant phase for the entire pupillary area, so that only when the pupils were very constricted could spherical aberration play a certain role. From this evidence it was clear that spherical aberration did not affect vision and that the quality of the image was not distorted (Y Le Grand).

In recent years, however, wavefront analysis using new aberrometers has confirmed the theoretical bases and experimental measurements of 50 years earlier.

RESULTS

On 2002, we treated mostly hyperopic patients, with PRK and a MEL 70 excimer laser. Results were encouraging, and continue to be so. The higher the hyperopia (3-4 diopters), with a highly hyperprolate final cornea, the better the near vision. The reach a good near vision, spherical aberration had to be made positive of 0.6-0.7 μm, regardless of initial curvature (Figs 12.15 and 12.16).

On 2003, despite modification of the photoablative program for myopic eyes, treatment with PRK/LASIK and MEL 70 excimer laser lead to better but still unsatisfactory results. As on February, 2004, we had treated 142 eyes—120 hyperopic, 20 myopic,

<table>
<tr><th colspan="2">PREOP</th><th>S.G.</th><th colspan="2">POSTOP 2 YEARS</th></tr>
<tr><td>BCVA</td><td>NEAR BCVA</td><td>56 years</td><td>UCVA</td><td>NEAR UCVA</td></tr>
<tr><td>+2.75 sph 10/10</td><td>+4.75 sph IJ</td><td>LEFT EYE</td><td>10/10</td><td>IJ</td></tr>
</table>

<table>
<tr><th rowspan="2">High order aberrations</th><th colspan="3">Zernike Polynomials</th><th rowspan="2">High order aberrations</th></tr>
<tr><th>Value</th><th>Zernike term</th><th>Value</th></tr>
<tr><td>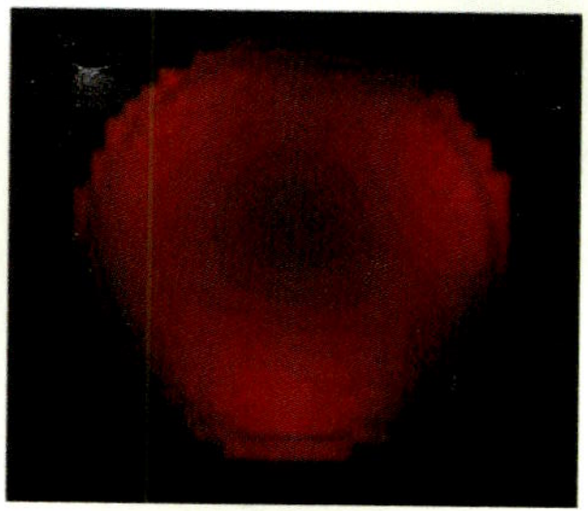</td><td>-0.337 µm</td><td>Z (4.0)</td><td>0.650 µm</td><td>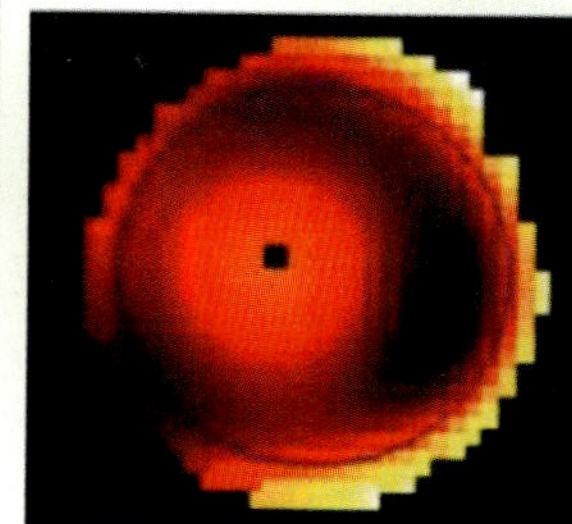</td></tr>
</table>

Fig. 12.15: Full correction of refractive defect for farsightedness. A major increase in spherical aberration *Z* (4.0) which changes from negative to positive. Pseudoaccommodation with near-sightedness / *J* without lenses

PREOP		MA	POSTOP	
BCVA	NEAR BCVA	60 years	UCVA	NEAR UCVA
+2.50 sph 10/10	+4.75 sph IJ	LEFT EYE	11/10	IJ

High order aberrations	Zernike Polynomials			High order aberrations
	Value	Zernike term	Value	
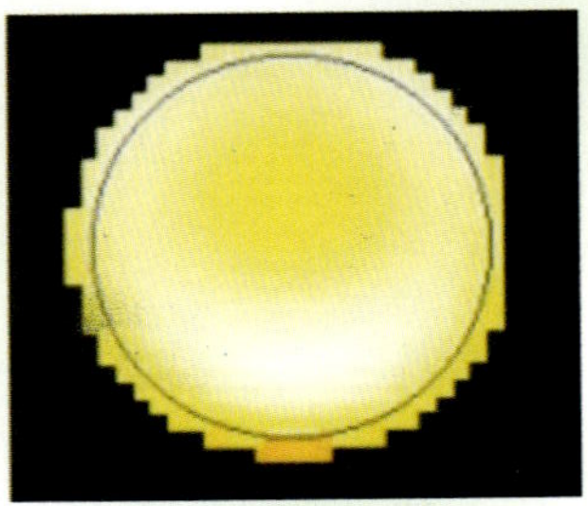	-0.483 µm	Z (4.0)	0.277 µm	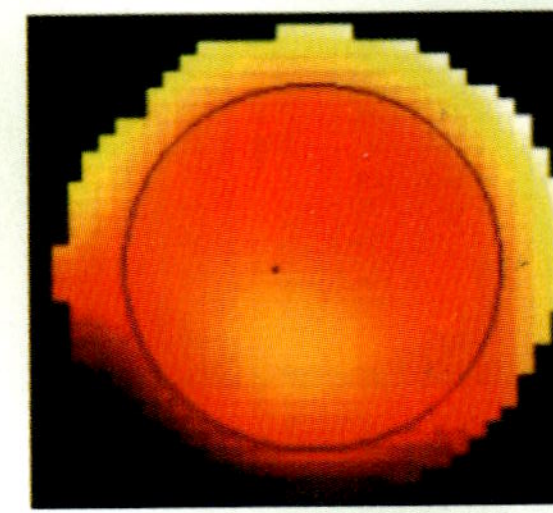

Fig. 12.16: MA 60 years. Full correction of refractive defect for farsightedness with an increase of 1/10 in vision. A major increase in spherical aberration *Z* (4.0) which changes from negative to positive. Pseudoaccommodation with near-sightedness *IJ* without lenses

2 emmetropes. On 2004 we adopted the MEL 80 excimer laser, capable of reaching a certain degrees of prolateness for low and medium myopia, and reached the target. It is easier to make hyperprolate a refracted cornea than an oblate cornea. This means making positive a spherical aberration not excessively negative. At the same time the mathematical calculations for refractive compensation, for unit of positivization of spherical aberration, became more precise, allowing a standardization of the technique.

In hyperopic eyes, positivization of spherical aberration had to be of 0.8 to 1.0 μm, with a refractive hypercorrection for compensation of 0.5 to 0.75 diopters. In presbyopic myopic eyes positivization of spherical aberration had to be of 1.1 to 1.2 μm, with a refractive hypocorrection of 2 to 2.5 diopters. This always considering the positivization (hyperops) or negativization (myops) induced by standard treatment.

From all these calculations, derived clearly the correction for the emmetrope: positivization of spherical aberration and refractive treatment for compensation. Single or compound astigmatism could be treated with the same rules defined for spherical defects, according to their sign.

From March 2004 to today, April 2005, we have treated a total of 128 eyes – 86 hyperops, 32 myops, 10 emmetropes. During the last year-and –half, Carl Zeiss Meditech in Germany started new experiments with MEL and CRS Master (Dieter Dausch, Eckard Schroder), with similar results. Furthermore, they could

PREOP		BP	POSTOP	
BCVA	NEAR BCVA	49 years	UCVA	NEAR UCVA
10/10 + 4 ph	+6.50 ph IJ	OS	10/10	I-II J

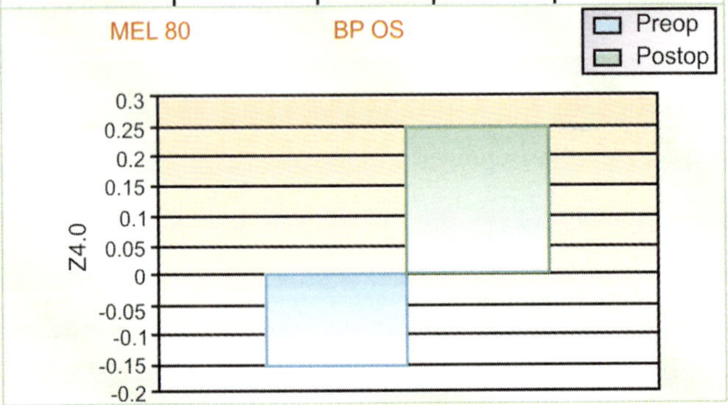

Fig. 12.17

highlight safety of treatment, without loss in contrast sensitivity at distant and close vision, no halos, etc.

A Few Examples with the MEL 80 Excimer Laser

Hyperopic patient of forty-eight-year-old, + 4.00 spherical (Figs 12.17 and 12.18). All refractive and aberrometric data reported, final refraction was satisfactory, and inversion of spherical aberration, turning from negative to positive. Topographical examination shows how the cornea becomes hyperprolate after the treatment.

Fifty-year-old myopic and astigmatic patient (Figs 12.19 and 12.20). Pre- and postoperative refractive and aberrometric data are presented, as well as the power

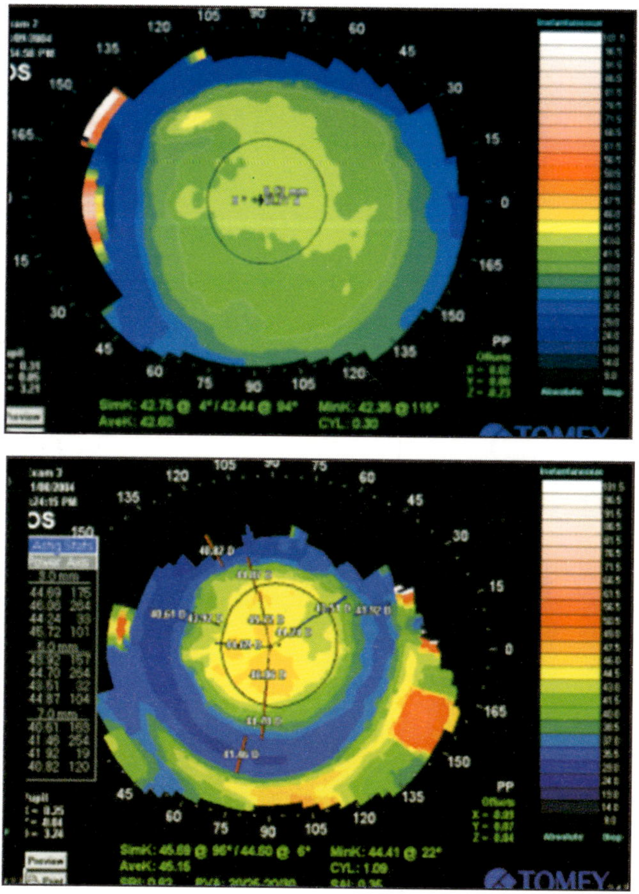

Fig. 12.18

difference map. Besides the good refractive result, both for distance and near vision, it is interesting to note how pre- and postoperative spherical aberration is quite similar and always negative. It is important to

PREOP		NF	POSTOP 6 MONTHS	
BCVA	NEAR BCVA	50 years	UCVA	NEAR UCVA
8-9/10 -6.00 sph; -3.00cyl 180°	1Δw -4.50 sph; -3.00 cyl 180°	OS	8-9/10	I Δw

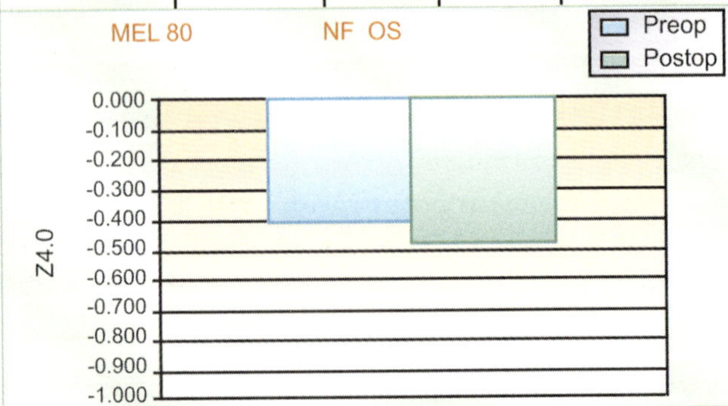

Fig. 12.19

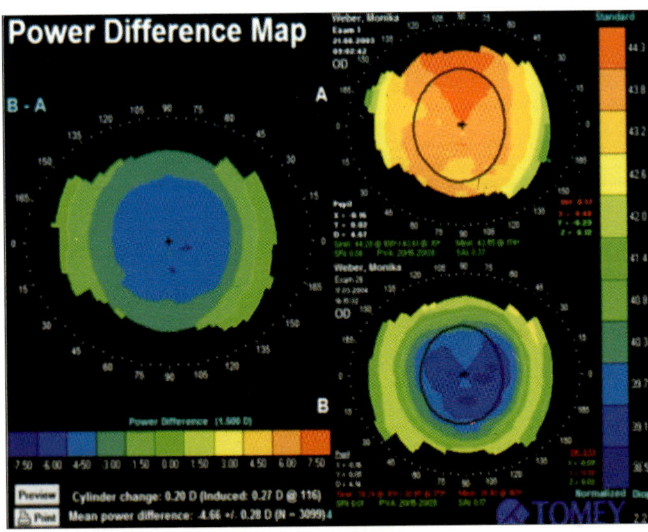

Fig. 12.20

remember, however, that without the positivization treatment (presbyopic correction), the simple refractive treatment would have induced a 2.5 times negative spherical aberration. This is very important in order to understand the results. Thus, when we talk about positivization, this does not mean only to achieve a positive spherical aberration, but even a substantially less negative one. Another interesting data: on topography, instantaneous algorithm, no sign of presbyopic correction can be perceived, meaning that no central island is observed.

Fifty-seven-year Old Emmetropic Patient (Figs 12.21 and 12.22)

As it almost always happens, emmetropia is a virtual reality. Usually, a small positive or seldom negative component is present, as in the case shown below. Refractive results for distance and near have been satisfactory, spherical aberration changed from negative to slightly positive. Postoperative corneal map shows the features of a hyperopic treatment, as always when treating emmetropic eyes.

During the last months, we started the treatment of pseudophakic eyes. Presently we have treated 8 of them , with refractive defects related to IOL miscalculation, and other problems.

Sixty-two-year-old pseudophakic patient (Fig. 12.23). Treatment is similar to that of a presbyopic,

PREOP PSEUDOFACHICO		SA	POSTOP 6 MONTHS	
BCVA	NEAR BCVA	57 years	UCVA	NEAR UCVA
10/10 -0.25 sph	1Δw +1.50 sph	OD	10/10	I Δw

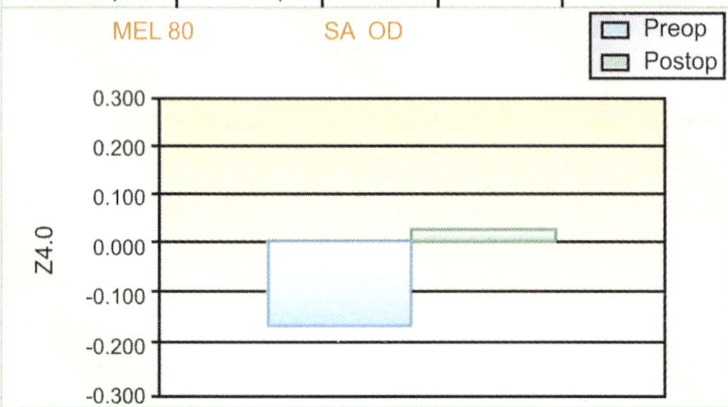

Fig. 12.21

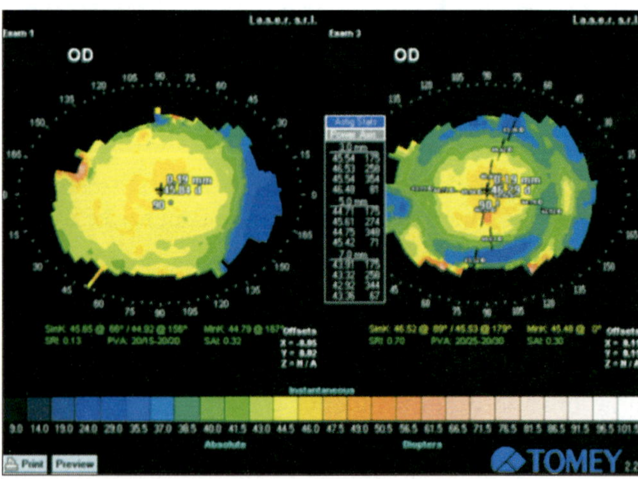

Fig. 12.22

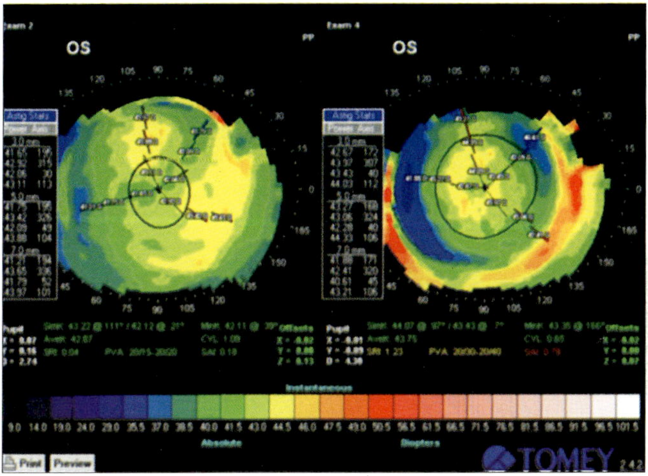

Fig. 12.23

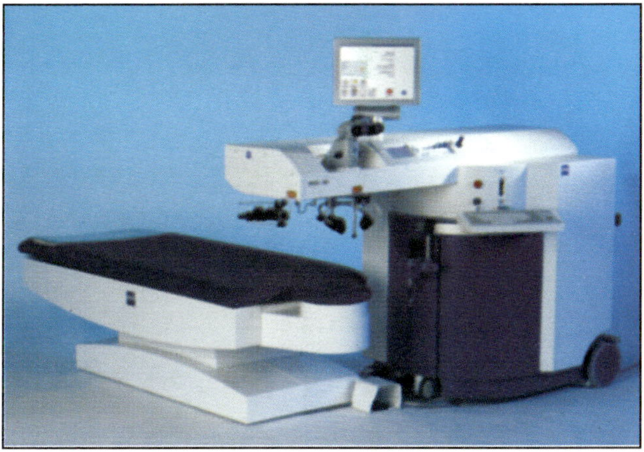

Fig. 12.24

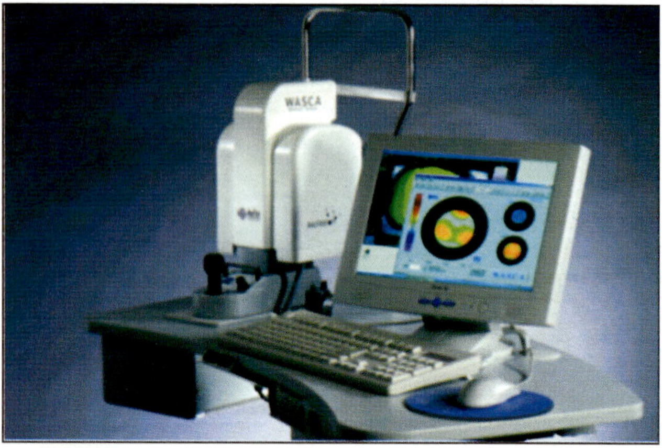

Fig. 12.25

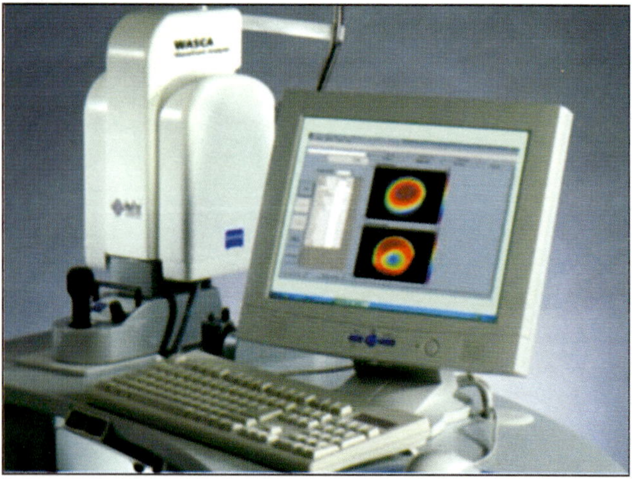

Fig. 12.26

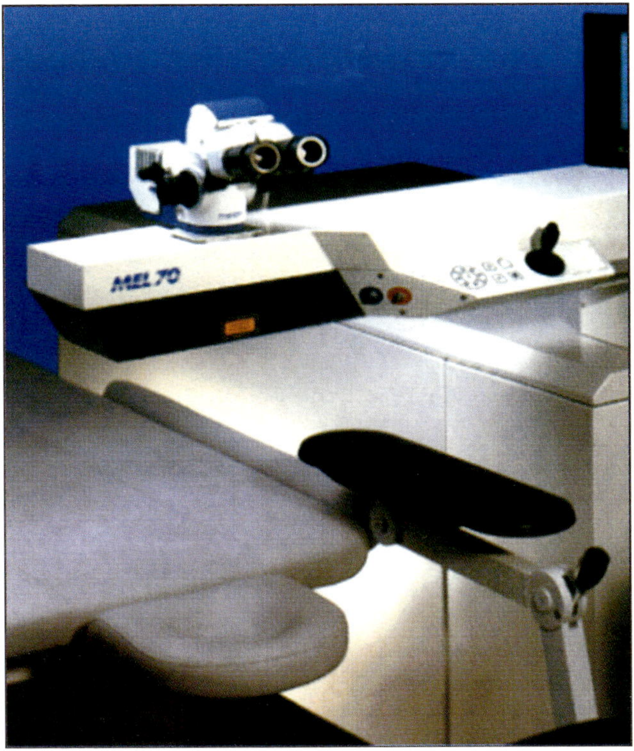

Fig. 12.27

phakic, hyperopic patient. Refractive and aberrometric results are similar, as well as topographic views.

The main interest in this technique is related to its possible alternative to pseudoaccommodative or diffractive IOLs for the correction of presbyopia. For the correction of IOL calculation error-derived refractive defects, the advantages are two-fold: the error is eliminated and the patient acquires near vision correction. After cataract surgery it can be utilized to restore near vision capabilities.

The latest development, still undergoing the experimental phase, concerns the making of corneal contact lenses for the correction of presbyopia, with the same scheme and analysis used for corneal treatment. Similar studies have been conducted in the past, without substantial results. Difficulties are manifold – i.e. ablation rate, different hydration if the contact lens is of the soft type, leons motion on the cornea, etc.). We are persuaded that presently most of these difficulties are solved, and the refractive results in the correction of presbyopia are really encouraging.

If these preliminary results would be confirmed, through the use of custom-made trial lenses, we could have the patient try the actual result of his possible refractive treatment.

BIBLIOGRAPHY

1. Agarwal A. Presbyopia. Slack Inc 2002.
2. Applegate RA, Thibos LN, Hilmantel G. "Optics of aberroscopy and super vision". J Cataract Refrac Surg 2001.
3. Artal P, Hoffer H, Williams DR, Aragon JL. Dynamic of ocularaberration during accomodation. Optical Society of America Annual Meeting 1999.
4. Bartoli F, Ipotesi di correzione aberrometrica della presbiopia. SOI 2002.
5. Bartoli F. Aberrometric correction of presbyopia. Refractive on-line 2004.

6. Bartoli F. Aberrometro ad alta definizione WASCA, link aberrometrico con Mel 70 G-Scan, The aberrometers. Fabiano 2002.
7. Bennett Arthur G, Rabbetts, Ronald B. Clinical Visual Optics 3e. Butterworth-Heinemann, 1998.
8. Born M, Wolf E. Principles of Optics 7e. Cambridge University Press, 1999.
9. Buratto L, Cantera E, Dal Fiume C, Genisi C, Merlin U, Topografia corneale. CAMO editore 1995.
10. Buratto L, Picardo V. Focal points in chirurgia rifrattiva. Fabiano 2001.
11. Burkhard Dick H, Werner T, Kaiser S, Wrede J. Dynamic wavefront measurements of eyes with accommodative IOL. 3rd Internationan congress of wavefront sensing and aberration-free refractive correction 2002.
12. Caimi F, La correzione laser dell'ipermetropia. Fabiano 2001.
13. Dausch D, Klein RJ, Schroeder E, Laserb ad eccimeri in oftalmologia. Medical Books 1992.
14. Dausch D, Lee S, Schroeder E, Wottke M. Wavefront Guided Correction of Presbyopia. 8th ESCRS Winter Meeting 2004.
15. Dick B, Goes F, Grabner G. The importance of resolution in aberrometry, ASCSRS-ASOA 2002.
16. Dossi F, Dossi R, Suppo E. Tecniche chirurgiche per la correzione dei difetti rifrattivi. Chirurgia rifrattiva, Fabiano 2000.
17. Geary, Joseph M. Introduction to wavefront sensing. SPIE Press, 1995.
18. Goodman, Joseph W. Fourier Optics 2e. McGraw-Hill, 1996.
19. Hecht, Eugene: Optics 3e. Addsion Wesley, 1997.
20. Le Grand Y. Optique physiologique,Revue d'optique. Paris 1956.
21. Liang J, Brimm B, Goelz S, Bille JF. "Objective measurement of wave aberrations of the human eye with the use of Hartmann-Shack wave-front sensor". J Opt Soc Am Acad 1994;11:1949-57.
22. Liuzzi L, Bartoli F, Manuale di Oftalmologia, ed. Minerva Medica 2002.

23. Machat JJ. Excimer laser refractive surgery, Slack Incorporated 1996.
24. Mahajan Virendra N. Optical Imaging and Aberrations, SPIE Press, 1998.
25. Mastropasqua L, Nubile M . "Lo studio delle aberrazioni oculari". L'oculista italiano No. 131 2001.
26. Miller Donald T. Retinal Imaging and Vision at the Frontiers of Adaptive Optics. Physics Today 2000;531,31.
27. Neal D, Copland J, Topa D, Vogelsang H, Bergt M. WaveFront Sciences/Asclepion Meditec WASCA: The technology, calibration, dynamic range, resolution, pecision and accuracy. The Aberrometers, Fabiano 2002.
28. Neal Daniel R, et al. Complete Light Analysis System User's Manual. WaveFront Sciences, May 1999.
29. Neal Daniel R, Hedlund E, Lederer M, Collier A, Spring C, Yanta W. Shack-Hartmann wavefront sensor testing of aero-optic phenomena, 20th AIAA Measurement and Ground Testing Technology Conference. June 1998.
30. Neal DR, Alford WJ, Gruetzner JK, "Amplitude and phase beam characterization using a two-dimensional wavefront sensor." SPIE 2870, 1996;72–82.
31. Neal DR, Armstrong DJ, Turner WT. "Wavefront sensors for control and process monitoring in optics manufacture." SPIE 2993 1997.
32. Pallikaris IG, Panagopoulu SI. Dynamic wavefront refractomy with asclepion aberrometer in the accommodation process. ASCSRS-ASOA 2002.
33. Piovella M, Camesasca FI, Kusa B. LASIK custom ablation based on WASCA aberrometry. Refractive on-line 2002.
34. Salmon T, West R, Kenmore T, Gasser W. "Evaluation of the COAS Shack-Hartmann Aberrometer as an Autorefractor." Optometry and Vision Science 2001;78(12):94.
35. Salz JJ. Chirurgia laser della cornea,Medical books 1996.
36. Schachar RA. Retinal imaging aberrometry. Ophtalmology 2002.
37. Smith, George, Atchison, David A. The Eye and Visual Optical Instruments. Cambridge University Press 1997.

38. Spadea L, Sabetti L, Bianco G, Santacroce B, Balestrazzi E. Standard vs wavefront-driven corneal ablation: Results of an intraindividual comparison. ASCRS 2002.
39. Thibos L, Hong X. "Clinical Applications of the Shack–Hartmann Aberrmeter." Optom Vis Sci 1999;76,817-25.
40. Vinciguerra P, Atlante di topografia corneale. Fogliazza editore 1995.

CHAPTER 13

Surgical Reversal of Presbyopia

Warren D Cross, Gene W Zdenek (USA)

INTRODUCTION

During the peak of the industrial revolution, there was a carpenter who invested much time and energy to develop his business reputation as a fine craftsman. A devastating accident nearly severed his hand and prevented him from continuing his most cherished woodworking occupation. He asked his friend if he could borrow money to start another business. His friend and future partner was only able to offer him \$ 26. With this initial investment, they started an optical laboratory to grind lenses for eyeglasses in Rochester, New York. They both helped grow a business that today generates \$ 2 to \$ 3 billion in annual revenue and employs over 13,000 employees in 35 countries. This business is still named after its two founders—Bausch and Lomb.

There is a modern-day analogy to the Bausch and Lomb story. It involves one very successful surgical ophthalmologist who was a pioneer in refractive eye surgery. An unfortunate accident permanently injured his right hand, ending his career as an ophthalmic surgeon. Rather than accepting this situation in a negative way, Ronald Schachar applied his high levels of energy, skills, and intelligence into diligently pursuing answers to one of the most perplexing questions that we have in ophthalmology today. What causes presbyopia? What can be done to reverse this process?

While an ophthalmology resident at the University of Chicago, Ronald A Schachar began questioning the validity of the Helmholtz's theory. The authors have personally observed his quest to answer these questions as an amazing course of events, experiments and discoveries since 1992.

One cannot begin to explain the cause of presbyopia and its subsequent treatment without first understanding the actual mechanism of accommodation. Schachar believed that the solution to treating presbyopia could be found in understanding the true mechanism of accommodation. So the odyssey began. This is how one tragic incident drove one individual ophthalmologist to begin solving the last refractive problem left in the present-day visual correction revolution, i.e. presbyopia.

Ever since 1677, when Descartes first observed the ability of the human eye to focus on objects at different distances in a visual field, the mechanism has fascinated and eluded physiologists and optical physicists. It was not until 1855, when Hermann von Helmholtz[1] learned that the central portion of the human lens thickened during accommodation that the mechanism of accommodation was theorized. From this observation, he concluded that contraction of the circular ciliary muscle produces relaxation of zonules, which reduces the tension on the zonule and allows the lens to increase its convexity. This mechanism of accommodation is an *active* contraction of the ciliary muscle that *passively* allows the change in the shape of the lens.

For over 140 years, this theory has been tested, analyzed and evaluated by physicists and physiologists alike. Hundreds of studies have been performed on the human lens, especially in conjunction with its ability to accommodate. These studies failed to explain many aspects of accommodation. Presbyopia, the progressive loss of accommodation with age, was attributed to sclerosis of the lens. The following explains the major observations that are found unexplained and inconsistent with the Helmholtz's theory.

INCONGRUENCIES IN THE HELMHOLTZ'S THEORY

The first and most compelling contradiction to Helmholtz's theory occurs when trying to apply the theory in order to make a deformable lens, similar to the young human crystalline lens, that can change optical power by approximately 10 diopters. *According to Helmholtz's theory, a small outward equatorial displacement of a deformable lens should produce a decrease in central optical power (Fig. 13.1). In fact, a small outward equatorial displacement produces a large increase in the central optical power of a deformable lens.*[15]

Spherical aberration is a common optical occurrence in all lenses. Spherical aberration increases when the central and peripheral curvatures of a given lens become steeper. Helmholtz's theory contends that both the central and peripheral lens convexity uniformly increase. In other words, the convexity of the entire lens

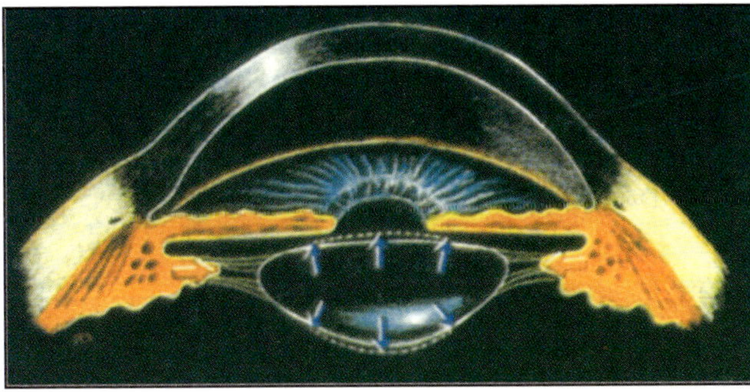

Fig. 13.1: Line drawing depicting Helmholtz's theory

during accommodation should become more uniform. The spherical aberration of a lens can be decreased if its convex surface is aspherical. There is more convexity to the central portion of the lens than there is to the peripheral portion of the lens. It has been clinically and experimentally shown that during accommodation, the human crystalline lens demonstrates less spherical aberration.[4,5] By the laws of optics, this can only occur if the convexity of the lens is becoming less uniformly convex, i.e. the convexity of the center of the lens is increasing while the convexity of the periphery is decreasing.

There is yet another perplexing problem with the theory of accommodation as explained by the Helmholtz's theory. This has been so baffling to physiologists and optical physicists that it has been named the "lens paradox". Attempts to explain this paradox have been fruitless.[7] Because the lens tissue is ectoderm, it continues to grow and its diameter increases approximately 20 microns/year.[6] As the crystalline lens grows in diameter, the optical power should increase. Emmetropes should progressively become myopic with presbyopia. During accommodation and gradually with age, there is a decrease in tension of the zonules according to Helmholtz. If this decrease in tension does occur, it should have two effects. First, the lens should passively accommodate, which would mean myopia would occur with presbyopia. Secondly, gravity should have more of an effect on the larger, heavier lens. In fact, our clinical experience with presbyopia is that patients become hyperopic.

The next observation that is inconsistent with Helmholtz's theory is the effect of gravity on the lens during accommodation.[3] In accordance with the Helmholtz's theory, during accommodation, gravitational forces should displace the lens. The reason for this belief is that with contraction of the ciliary muscle (causing a relaxation of the zonules), the lens should then be less stable in the eye and, therefore, should be able to shift with gravity. A well-constructed experiment by Schachar in 1994[3] clearly shows that there is no effect of gravity on the young accommodating crystalline lens. In 1998, when a 76-year-old presbyopic John Glenn re-entered outer space, no change in his spectacle correction was required. There was clearly no shift in the lens position of his crystalline lens in a weightless environment.

A very reasonable deduction from the Helmholtz's theory is that if there were an anterior disinsertion of the ciliary muscle, the eye should automatically lose accommodation and become myopic. To verify this corollary, an experiment was conducted in which the anterior ciliary muscle of primates was disinserted. There was a loss of accommodation, with hyperopia as opposed to the anticipated myopia.[8]

If the lens was, in fact, preventing accommodation because of sclerosis, then the circular muscle fibers, which are largely responsible for accommodation, should atrophy. Histological examination of the circular muscle fibers by Tamm et al clearly shows that just the opposite occurs.[9]

With the Helmholtz's theory in mind, our belief has been that presbyopia is caused by sclerosing[2] or stiffening of the lens, preventing it from passively becoming more spherical. The disease of presbyopia, which occurs as a result of the decline in the amplitude of accommodation, is a process that occurs with stunning predictability throughout life for generations and is independent of genetics, environmental pressures or color (Fig. 13.2). A simple question must be asked: *What disease known to man exists that can be predicted in 100 percent of the population within one and a half years of a given age?*

It is these compelling discrepancies and inconsistencies in the Helmholtz's theory that have driven ophthalmologists to answer these paradoxical questions.

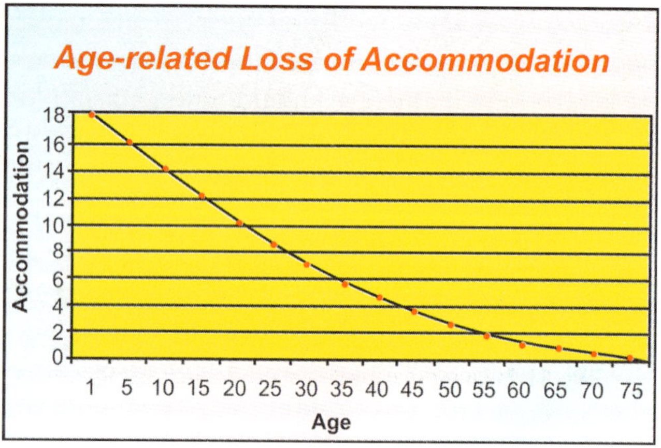

Fig. 13.2: Age-related loss of accommodation graph: The close relationship presbyopia has to age contradicts the Helmholtz's theory. Presbyopia could not possibly be the result of a lens sclerosing disease

To explain the deficiencies or inconsistencies in Helmholtz's theory of accommodation and to further refine the definition and cause of presbyopia, Schachar began his long journey to develop a new theory for the mechanism of accommodation. His new theory[10-15] states that the human crystalline lens is under increased tension equatorially during accommodation as opposed to decreased tension. It is the anterior radial muscle fibers of the ciliary muscle that arch towards the sclera during accommodation. This is the reason why the anterior radial muscle fibers atrophy following presbyopia. This arching increases the tension on the equatorial zonules, leaving the anterior and posterior

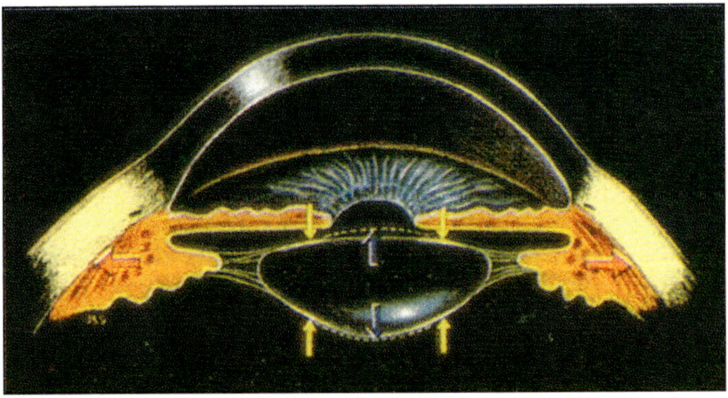

Fig. 13.3: Line drawing depicting Schachar's theory

zonules more relaxed. The anterior and posterior zonules are allowed to relax, because the posterior longitudinal and posterior radial muscle fibers move anteriorly. The tension that the equatorial zonules place on the equator of the human crystalline lens produces a central steepening along with a peripheral flattening of the lens during accommodation (Fig. 13.3).

This clearly explains why spherical aberration decreases during accommodation. Schachar very eloquently demonstrates this central steepening and peripheral flattening of a deformable biconvex lens when he pulls on the equator of a biconvex air-filled *Mylar* balloon (Figs 13.4A to 13.5B).[16] The reflections of a person's face in this balloon reflect the evidence that there is central steepening and peripheral flattening of this convex surface.

If the Helmholtz's theory were valid, one should be able to construct a bionic version of an accommodating

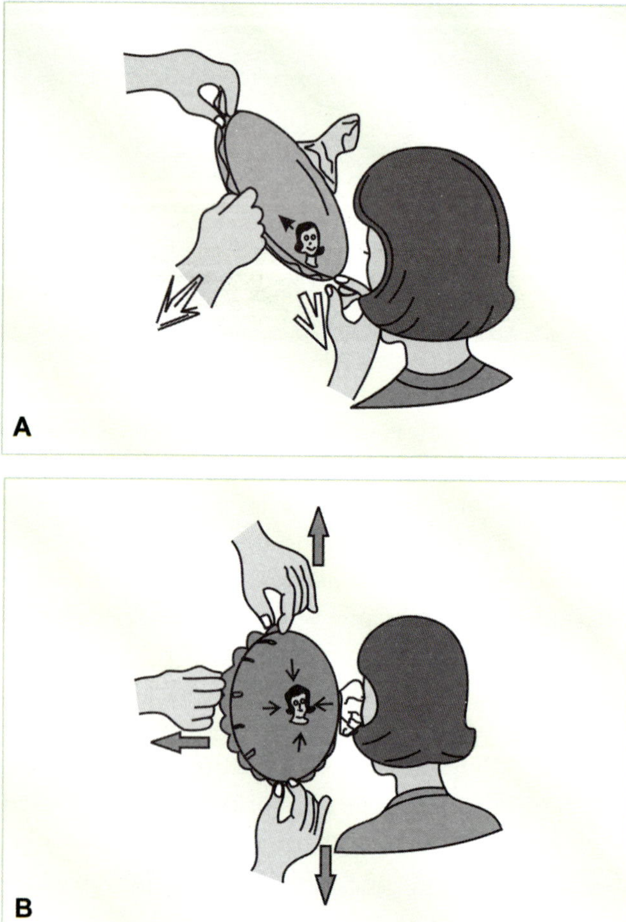

Figs 13.4A and B: Line drawings of Mylar balloon with patient: **(A)** Look at your reflection in the center of an air-filled Mylar balloon, and **(B)** Note that your reflection in the center of the balloon minifies when the balloon's equator is stretched. This demonstrates that the center of the balloon is steepening with the equatorial stretching

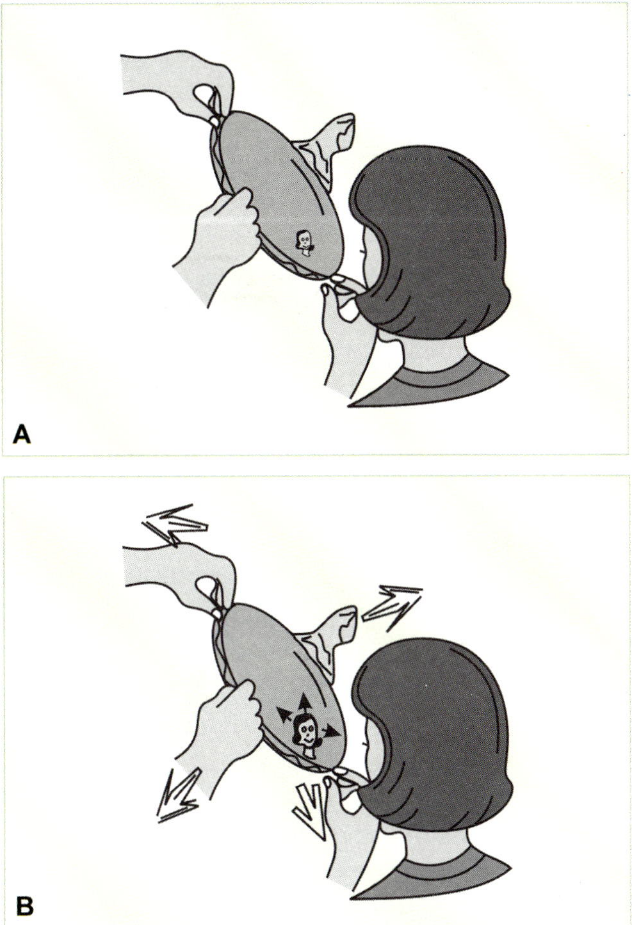

Figs 13.5A and B: Line drawings of Mylar balloon: **(A)** Then look at your reflection in the periphery of the Mylar balloon, and **(B)** Note that your reflection in the periphery of the balloon enlarges when the balloon's equator is stretched. This demonstrates that the periphery of the balloon is flattening while the center is steepening when the balloon's equator is stretched (Courtesy: R Schachar)

lens. This task has eluded researchers ever since Helmholtz's theory was postulated. A very strong validation of Schachar's new theory of accommodation is that he has, for the first time in history, successfully constructed a single-element, variable-focused lens that can change optical power to the order of 10 diopters.[14] This is accomplished by simply applying a small outward radial force to the equator of a deformable lens.[15]

Schachar's theory of accommodation goes well beyond the ophthalmic community. The validity of the Schachar theory of accommodation is further demonstrated by the fact that it can be applied to many different areas, both familiar and unfamiliar to us, as ophthalmic surgeons. The authors would refer you to his original article in the *Annals of Ophthalmology* of 1999,[15] where he discusses the implication that his theory has on ocean tides, magnetic fluids and even the shape of galaxies. An amazing accomplishment for one individual! It is interesting to compare the mechanisms that are proposed by the Helmholtz's theory of accommodation to what we, as surgeons, know about changes of the cornea after surgery. The Helmholtz's theory states that if the zonules are put on tension, the center and periphery of the lens flattens. Ever since ophthalmologists began suturing cataract incisions, we have unknowingly been observing and using Schachar's theory of lens deformation. If Helmholtz's theory were correct, a tight 12 o'clock suture on a cataract incision should cause central and peripheral corneal flattening in that meridian. We all know that this is not the case. When sutures are placed too tightly in a surgical incision, both slit-lamp and topographical examination reveal flattening of the peripheral cornea and adjacent sclera. The central portion of the cornea becomes steeper in that meridian. With a tight stitch at 12 o'clock, the astigmatism occurs "with-the-rule (WTR)". This is the most common clinical verification of Schachar's theory.

When a spherical object is pulled or has increased tension circumferentially, the central portion of the spherical object becomes steeper, and the peripheral portions of the spherical object become flatter. With the new Schachar theory now in place, we can begin to examine the many possibilities for reversing presbyopia, and three methods become theoretically apparent:

- Stopping the growth of the crystalline lens (20 microns/year)
- Shrinking the length of the equatorial zonules in order to increase their tension
- Increasing the ciliolenticular space between the ciliary muscle and the equator of the lens. This would then indirectly increase the tension on the equatorial zonules by putting them on stretch.

As one can see, any one or combination of these three mechanisms can lead to the reversal or prevention of presbyopia. *Due to technological limitations, we currently neither are able to stop the growth of the lens nor can we shrink the equatorial zonules. For these reasons, the only plausible reversal of presbyopia is an expansion of the space between the ciliary muscle and the equator of the crystalline lens. This is known as scleral expansion.*

Radial sclerotomies to produce scleral expansion were first described by Schachar.[25] It has recently been popularized by a multicenter study headed by Spencer Thornton. It appears that early results of radial sclerotomy (either by diamond knife or by excimer laser) yield less than 3 diopters of restored accommodation and the effect decreases with time, often within months. This is still an area of active research and supports Schachar's theory of accommodation.

SUMMARY OF SCHACHAR'S THEORY OF ACCOMMODATION

Presbyopia is due to normal equatorial lens growth, which interferes with the normal function of the ciliary muscle. Scanning microscopy has shown that there are three types of zonules: anterior, equatorial and posterior. During accommodation, the anterior and posterior zonules appear to relax. The equatorial zonules have separate and distinct insertions into the ciliary body. With age, the anterior and posterior zonules move further from the crystalline lens equator so that even though the equator is enlarging, stability is maintained with increasing age. During accommodation, the equatorial zonules transmit ciliary muscle contraction to increase the tension on the equator of the crystalline lens. The peripheral one-third of the crystalline lens flattens, while the center steepens, thus, increasing its central optical power. With increasing age, the distance between the crystalline lens equator and the ciliary muscle decreases. The amount of stretch on the anterior radial ciliary muscle fibers is reduced, and decreases the amount of force which can be applied to the crystalline lens equator. Accommodation becomes increasingly difficult, then progressively impossible with age, resulting in presbyopia.

The current technique for surgical reversal of presbyopia (SRP) is scleral expansion. This technique involves re-establishing the physiological space between the lens equator and the ciliary muscle. Once the anterior ciliary muscle fibers are stretched, accommodation begins immediately and improves over several months as the muscles regain their strength.[10-13,17]

THE HISTORY, DEVELOPMENT, PROBLEMS AND RESULTS OF THE SCLERAL EXPANSION BAND

1971–1992

- Theory and testing on animal and cadaver eyes with trials of radial and zigzag scleral incisions. Scleral incisions were a very bloody procedure that was cosmetically unacceptable.
- The procedure produced slight amounts of increased accommodation (0.50–1.50 diopters).

- This surgically acquired accommodation was determined to regress at a faster rate than associated with physiological aging. The faster rate of regression was more related to scleral healing and contraction of fibers.

1992

- In Monterrey Mexico, Schachar,[12] Jose de la Garza Viejo,[18] and Antonio Garza, performed the first scleral expansion surgeries using hand-made polymethylmethacrylate (PMMA) encircling scleral expansion bands (SEBs).
- The bands had 16 equally spaced holes placed centrally in the 2 mm wide bands. A fornix-based 360-degree peritomy was used. The band was sutured to the sclera using 6-0 Mersilene sutures. A total of six eyes in six presbyopic patients underwent the surgery.
- Postoperatively, the six patients' results ranged from 5.8 to 11.1 D of accommodation.
- The suture cheese-wired through the fornix-based conjunctival flaps.
- SEBs were removed from one to three months postoperatively.

1992–1993

- The SEBs were then injection molded to ensure that they were smooth. A special order 6-0 clear Prolene suture from Ethicon was developed to attach the SEB to the sclera.

1993–1994

- Multiple presbyopic patients had SEB surgery under the auspices of an Institutional Review Board (IRB) in Houston by Warren D Cross, MD.[19] All patients experienced improvement in accommodation ranging from 1.5 to 12 D.
- All patients underwent a 6 mm 360-degree limbus-based peritomy. Using a specially developed caliper, scleral diameters were measured allowing the multiple sized bands to be custom fitted to the globe. SEB was attached using a continuous running Prolene suture with a knot buried under the band. The conjunctiva was meticulously closed using a horizontal running mattress suture.
- Five bands were removed within three days because of an acute increase in intraocular pressure (IOP) secondary to tight sutures.
- Additional bands were removed over the next 14 months because of conjunctival erosion secondary to knot placement.
- One band was removed before cataract surgery in a patient who developed bilateral posterior subcapsular cataracts (not related to the unilateral band application).
- The first two original patients continue to have their bands in place 6 years later. The effect on accommodation has decreased with age but is still measurable. Both are cosmetically acceptable. The first patient (SH) age 59, six years postoperatively

had at least 1.75 D of accommodation, requiring +0.25 add over distance correction to read J_1 at 40 cm (Fig. 13.6). The world's second patient (KH) age 48 at six years postoperative read J_1 at 40 cm without an add (Fig. 13.7). Both patients had normal IOPs.

1994–1996

- Multiple SEB prototypes are developed and tested by Schachar, Cross[19] and Richard Yee,[20] to avoid the

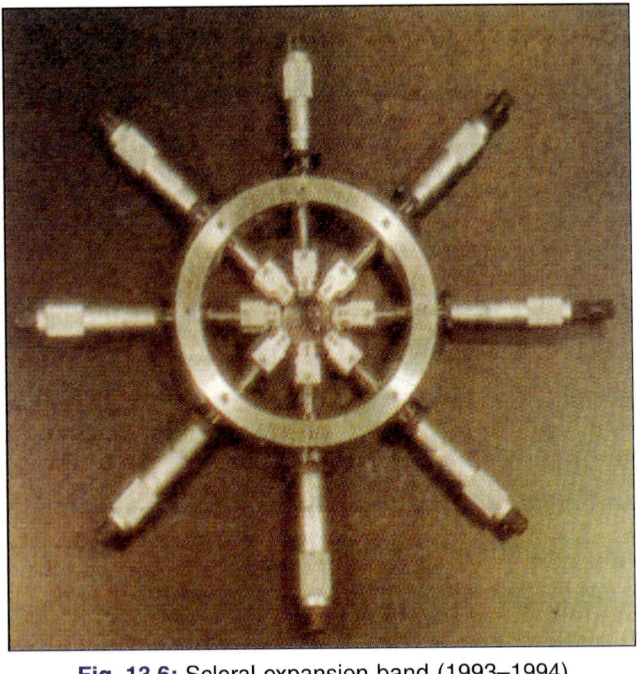

Fig. 13.6: Scleral expansion band (1993–1994)

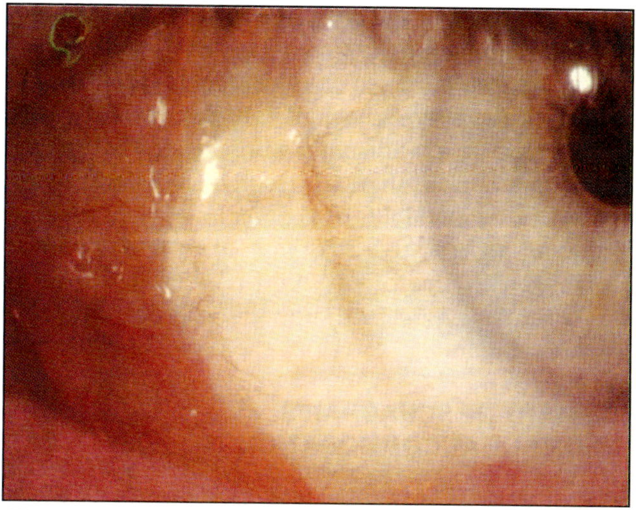

Fig. 13.7: Close-up of scleral band, six years postoperative [(SH) Courtesy: Warren Cross]

use of sutures. Prototypes used steel and titanium SEBs with adjustable clips that were micromachined by IBM. The concept was that the size of the band could be adjusted like the clips of a hatband. The metal SEB prototypes could not be safely passed around the eye even when viscoelastics, mineral oil or special surfactants were used.

- The metal SEB prototypes were abandoned.

1996–1997

- Instead of an encircling band, a SEB prototype is made consisting of four individual PMMA sections. Each section of the SEB is passed through scleral belt loops (sutureless), overlapped and then fused while on the eye using a specially designed microsized ultrasonic fusing device.

- The ultrasonic fusing device had a 2 mm square tip. The individual sections were overlapped and placed between a footplate and the ultrasonic fusing tip. Using hand pressure, the ultrasound was applied to produce fusion of each section.
- The band could now be custom fitted to the size of the globe and no sutures were needed to attach the band to the sclera.

1996

In Monterrey, Mexico, Viejo,[18] Cross,[19] and Yee,[20] performed the first SEB surgery passing the four individual sections of the band through 4 scleral belt loops using the individual overlapping sections and the hand-driven 2 mm tip ultrasonic device.

- The patient obtained approximately six diopters of accommodation
- Larry Lothringer, MD independently observed and verified these results
- The ultrasonically welded joints in the band were too rough and ultimately the band was removed because of recurrent conjunctival erosion problems
- At the University of Texas Medical Branch, Houston, under the auspices of an IRB, Yee,[20] with Cross[19] performed SEB surgery on six patients using individual segments, which were overlapped and fused with the ultrasonic device

- The fusion sites were smoothed with a special diamond and carbide dental drill. The four belt loops were placed along the 6:00, 9:00, 12:00, and 3:00 meridians. The fusion sites were not smooth enough and five of the SEBs were removed
- The patient with the remaining band continues to do well and has good accommodation
- Three additional patients had SEBs, but the belt loops were made thicker, i.e. the scleral dissection was deeper. The three patients developed anterior segment ischemia and the bands were immediately removed. None of these patients lost vision or had a change in their refraction.

1997

- The SEB segments were modified to have a tongue and groove junction
- The ultrasonic handpiece was modified to have a 1 mm, air pressure controlled tip in order to ensure a constant force during the fusion process. The time and force applied during the fusion process was automatically controlled
- The smoothing device was further refined
- All scleral belt loops are made along the 45° meridians
- In Marseilles, France, Jean Pierre Maistre,[21] Cross,[19] and Les Schachar, performed the new SEB procedure using the new prototype and the new ultrasonic device

- This center is established as the initial European testing center
- In Bangkok, Thailand, Ekkett Chansue, and L Schachar, performed scleral expansion with this new prototype and equipment, which established the first Asian center for presbyopia study
- In Puerta Vallarta, Mexico, Monica Gomez, Robert Epstein, and L Schachar, performed scleral expansion with the new prototype and new ultrasonic device
- In Recefe, Brazil, Heraldo Martins, and L Schachar performed scleral expansion with the new system
- All patients in the above new system had an increase in their amplitude of accommodation; but in some of the patients, there was still a problem with conjunctival erosion. There have also been occasional episodes of anterior segment ischemia requiring removal of the SEB.

1998

- In an attempt to prevent the anterior segment ischemic syndrome problems and to simplify and decrease instrumentation cost, a new prototype was developed
- The new design consisted of four individual PMMA segments, which were not connected to each other. The segments were placed in scleral belt loops along the 45° meridians
- Initial segments were 7 mm long, 1.2 mm wide and had ridges on the superior surfaces to enhance the

scleral lift. The segments were inserted into 2 mm wide, 5 mm long scleral belt loops

- The segments were tested in Monterrey, Mexico by Viejo,[18] at the first inaugural "surgical reversal of presbyopia" course. The following Ophthalmologists were in attendance and independently observed and evaluated patients pre- and postoperatively:
  - — Frank J Grady, Texas
  - — Sheldon Herzig, Canada
  - — Frederic B Kremer, Pennsylvania
  - — Larry Lothringer, Texas
  - — Howard N Straub, Colorado
  - — William W Waugh, Minnesota
  - — Gene W Zdenek, California
- The increased technical ease of the surgery and the postoperative accommodation results were excellent. These segments were too long and showed signs of sector anterior ischemia
- The scleral belt loops were narrowed to 900 microns wide and 4.0 mm in length
- Jean Pierre Maistre is the first European ophthalmologist to perform SRP; and Gene W Zdenek[22] was the first ophthalmologist to perform SRP on the first US patient in Mexico utilizing the current SEB segments and technique in February 1998
- In Recefe, Brazil, Heraldo Martins, and L Schachar performed scleral expansion with the new system. The first postoperative LASIK patient underwent successful SEB surgery

- Zdenek and Maistre modified the technique and instruments to shorten the total surgical time to approximately 30 minutes
- Sheldon Herzig is the first Canadian surgeon to perform SRP and began the process for SRP approval in Canada
- Lothringer performed SRP on two patients that were postoperative photorefractive keratectomies (PRKs)
- Zdenek did SRP on a patient with primary open-angle glaucoma producing a 12 mm decrease in IOP
- Marmer performed the first bilateral SEB in an ocular hypertensive patient with excellent results of a 10 mm decrease in IOP.

1999

- The SEB segments are modified dimensionally in order to increase the amplitude of accommodation and enhance segment stability
- US-FDA clinical trials begin phase I studies in six academic programs
- Cross begins international clinical trials evaluating SRP for treatment of primary ocular hypertension and primary open-angle glaucoma.

SURGICAL REVERSAL OF PRESBYOPIA (SRP)

Patient Selection

Indications for the Ideal Surgical Candidate

- 40 to 70 years old

- No refractive error at distance
- Binocular vision
- Less than +1.00 of hyperopia
- Hyperopes are more likely to require bilateral SRP.

Relative Contraindications

- LASIK following SRP. Conjunctival irregularities following SRP may interfere with the suction ring placement. Some successful LASIK procedures following SRP have been performed without difficulty.
- Monocular patient. This is pertinent only because of the investigational status of SRP.
- Patients beyond 70 years of age should be informed of the possibility of ciliary muscle atrophy.
- Severe keratoconjunctivitis Sicca. Appropriate management of this condition should be conducted prior to SRP. This may include lid hygiene, punctal occlusion or topical cyclosporine treatment.[19]
- Diabetes—insulin dependent or poorly controlled.
- Patients with hyperopia greater than +1.00 should have surgical correction prior to SRP. Whenever patients have pre-existing hyperopia, a significant amount of their accommodative ability is used for better vision at distance. Therefore, less of their accommodative amplitude gained by SRP is available for near vision.

Contraindications

- Previous cataract extraction
- Scleromalacia

- Previous trabeculectomy
- Coagulopathies
- Collagen vascular diseases.

Surgical Technique

Patient Preparation

Half percent proparacaine is instilled and the 12 o'clock position of the eye is marked at the slit- lamp. The patient is taken into the operating room and is prepped and draped in the usual sterile manner for intraocular surgery.

Quadrant Marking

A circular ring marker is used to accurately mark the four oblique axes.

Corneal Shield

A viscous lubricant is placed on the corneal shield which is then placed on the cornea to preserve the epithelium, ensure patient comfort, and an immediate improvement in postoperative near visual acuity.

Anesthesia

Four percent xylocaine is applied with a pledget spear to the quadrant to be operated. It is preferred to start with the inferior quadrants to avoid conjunctival edema that tends to develop towards the end of the case.

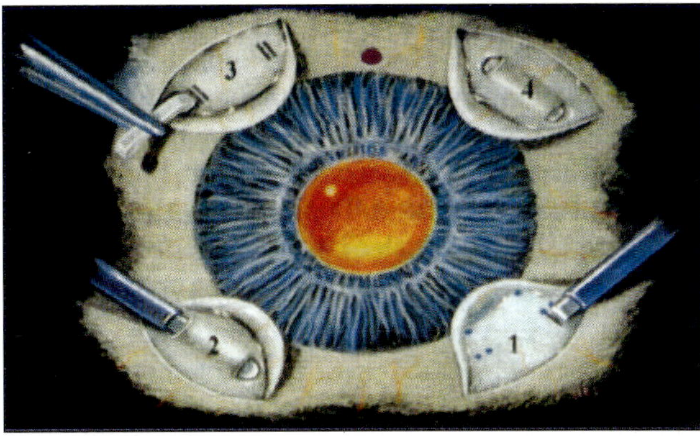

Fig. 13.8: Four general steps to surgical reversal of presbyopia (SRP) drawing: Step 1—sclerotomy, step 2—belt loop formation, step 3—insertion of SEB segment, and step 4—conjunctival closure

Conjunctival Opening

If large vessels are present, light conjunctival cautery should be used prior to making the incision. This incision is arcuate and lies 6 mm posterior to the limbus. This is dissected anteriorly up to 2 mm posterior to the limbus. Care should be taken not to disturb the 2 mm of sclera just posterior to the surgical limbus (Fig. 13.8). This area of the sclera for all four quadrants is the virgin territory. It should not be cauterized or grasped with any instruments to preserve its structural integrity. This area provides the scleral lift (Fig. 13.9).

Cautery

Scleral cautery should be kept at a minimal to avoid damage or shrinkage. Only the sclerotomy site can be lightly cauterized if necessary.

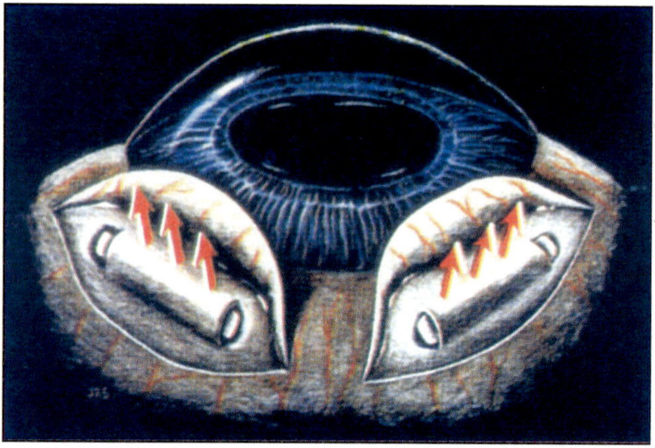

Fig. 13.9: Line drawing depicting vector forces in surgical reversal of presbyopia (SRP)

Scleral Marking

A specially designed four-pronged instrument is placed on the surgical limbus and rocked posteriorly to place two marks 2.75 mm posterior to the limbus and separated by 4.0 mm (Fig. 13.10).

Sclerotomy

A special preset diamond blade is used to make two sclerotomies 300 microns deep and 1.5 mm in length. This pair of sclerotomies are parallel to each other and *not* radial to the limbus. If the distance between the sclerotomies is too short, there will be less scleral lift. Conversely, if the distance is too great or the sclerotomies are not parallel, the SEB segment will not be sitting on full-thickness sclera. This will lead to segment instability.

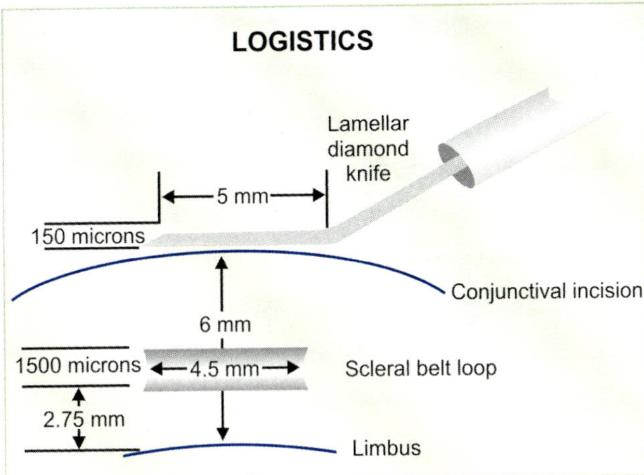

Fig. 13.10: Logistics graphic

Scleral Belt Loop Formation

A custom-designed long thin lamella diamond sclerotomy knife is used to make a scleral belt loop. Scleral fixation is achieved using a small two-pronged scleral twist pick. *This should not be placed anterior to the segment position to avoid damage to this region of the sclera. A surgical pearl here is that the correct depth of the belt loop is attained when there is a slight bulge of the diamond blade apparent under the sclera. The surgeon is too shallow when the actual blade can be seen through the sclera but too deep (Fig. 13.11) if no scleral bulge is seen.*

SEB Segment Insertion

Place a drop of saline in the SEB segment case to avoid losing the segment because of static electricity. A fine, nonlocking

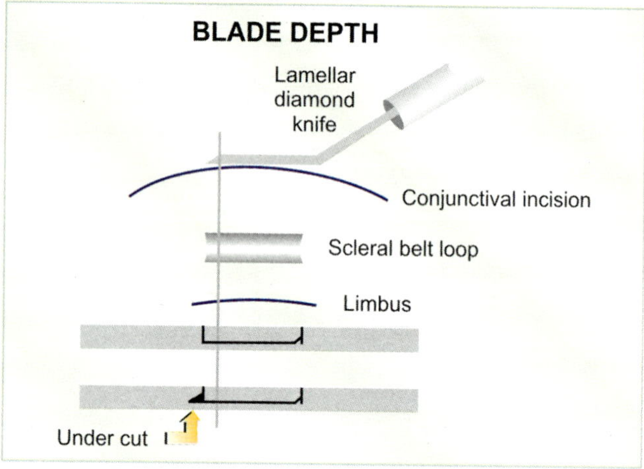

Fig. 13.11: Blade depth graphic: The vertical white line shows that the cutting edge of the knife is actually more advanced than one thinks. To avoid an "under cut" tilt the knife tip upward before reaching the exit scleral punch

needle holder is used to grasp the segment at its midpoint, flat bottom down. The SEB segment is then inserted into the *exit* side of the belt loop (Figs 13.12A and B). *The SEB segment is inserted in this direction to avoid irregular pockets/ridges within the belt loop*. The SEB segment is now centered within the belt loop to assure that the ends of the segment are protruding equally from both ends of the belt loop.

Conjunctival Closure

This is best performed using the same meticulous considerations we use when closing the conjunctiva over a trabeculectomy site. There can be no button

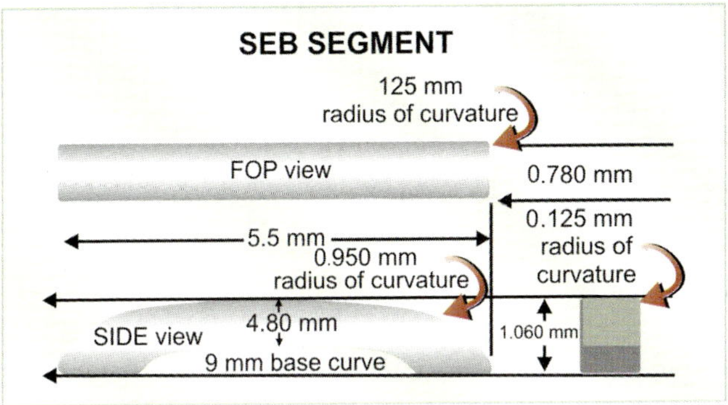

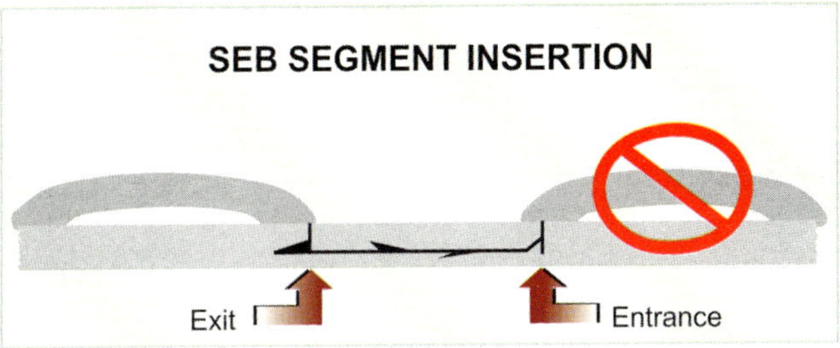

Figs 13.12A and B: SEB segment and insertion graphic: Remember, beginners, if the blade advancement through the scleral belt loop was not smooth and even, the SEB segment should be inserted through the belt loop exit first

holes, tears or gaps when approximating the conjunctiva. *This is the longest and the most critical part of the procedure.*

Mannitol

Just prior to finishing the last quadrant, 500 cc of intravenous 20 percent mannitol is started. This procedure will avoid the possibility of malignant glaucoma, which is theoretically possible but has never been reported in over 200 cases using the SEB segment technique.

Medications

After removing the protective corneal cover, instill pilocarpine 2 percent followed by an antibiotic/anti-inflammatory combination. It is imperative that the pupil is carefully observed for its ability to constrict in its normal symmetrical fashion. A pressure patch is then applied (optional). Extra strength acetaminophen or nonsteroidal anti-inflammatory drugs (NSAIDs) may be given if needed for any discomfort.

Postoperative Care

Postoperative Examination

On the first postoperative day, a thorough slit-lamp examination should be performed including a measurement of IOP. Of particular importance is observing symmetrical pupillary constriction and/or normal pupillary reaction, and flawless conjunctival closure. Any conjunctival defect should be surgically addressed at this time.

Medications

The patient should be started on topical antibiotic and anti-inflammatory eyedrops for two to three weeks. Initially, there is a transient decrease in goblet cell function due to conjunctival swelling. Therefore, it is very important to emphasize liberal use of artificial tears.

Exercises

We instruct our patients to practice reading daily in order to enhance/restore accommodation. Near-far ductions aid in rehabilitating the disuse atrophy present in some older patients. Conscious stimulation of the accommodation-convergence complex is felt to lead to a more efficient restoration of AC/A ratios.

Suture Removal

Sutures should never be removed sooner than 7 to 10 days postoperatively. Sutures are to be removed as dictated by patient's symptoms if necessary after the initial 10 days period.

Typical Patient Symptoms

- Very mild brow ache occurs frequently within the first 24 hours.
- Accommodative sclerolmyalgia was first described by Zdenek to explain the unique cluster of intermittent postoperative symptoms that are experienced by these patients during accommodation. This most often occurs without photophobia or lacrimation and is different from ciliary spasm. When the patients focuse at near, they experience clear vision but experience an associated ocular discomfort.

- Intermittent blurry near vision is common for the first 2 to 3 weeks following surgery. This is ordinarily caused by disruption of the tear film, and very rarely by transient corneal astigmatism induced by conjunctival swelling.
- Photosensitivity is experienced by many and is due to the tear film insufficiency. This resolves within two weeks.
- Accommodative fatigue occurs variably with patients for up to four to six weeks.
- Subconjunctival hemorrhage is quite obvious and should be part of the preoperative discussion with the patient. This resolves like any other subconjunctival hemorrhage.
- Minor, localized conjunctival hyperemia is present over the SEB segment for up to eight weeks.

Early Clinical Results

Accommodation has increased in all of the 200 patients who have undergone the surgical reversal of presbyopia (SRP). The documented increased range of accommodation varies from a minimum of +1.00 diopter up to +10.00 diopters. Perhaps, the most interesting phenomenon to occur with this procedure is the effect on the unoperated eye. The accommodation in the fellow eye improves by approximately 20 to 50 percent of what is measured in the operated eye. This unexpected benefit is probably explained by a central

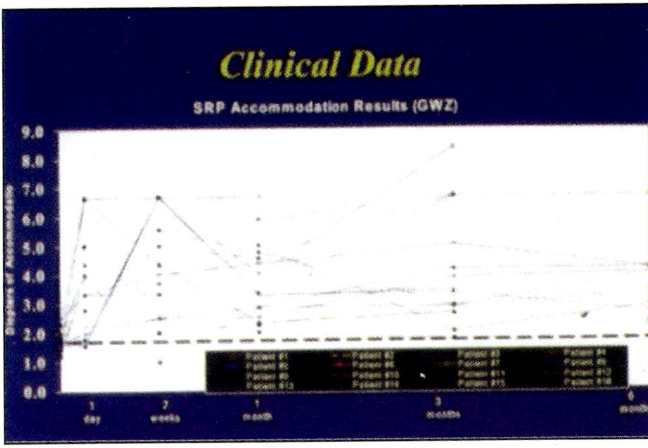

Fig. 13.13: Surgical reversal of presbyopia (SRP) accommodation results (Courtesy: Gene W Zdenek)

nervous system (CNS) mechanism transmitted via the Edinger-Westphal nucleus. Below are the results of the three largest studies using the current technique (Fig. 13.13). All measures of near point of accommodation were taken with the distance manifest correction in place.

Figure 13.14 represents the first 14 SRP procedures performed from February 98 to August 98. This represents 16 eyes (two bilateral cases), 8 females and 6 males ranging in age from 45 to 63 years, averaging 52 years of age. The horizontal dashed line represents the average preoperative baseline accommodation. Note the sporadic range of accommodation in the first postoperative month. Also, note the stabilization of accommodation by the sixth month.

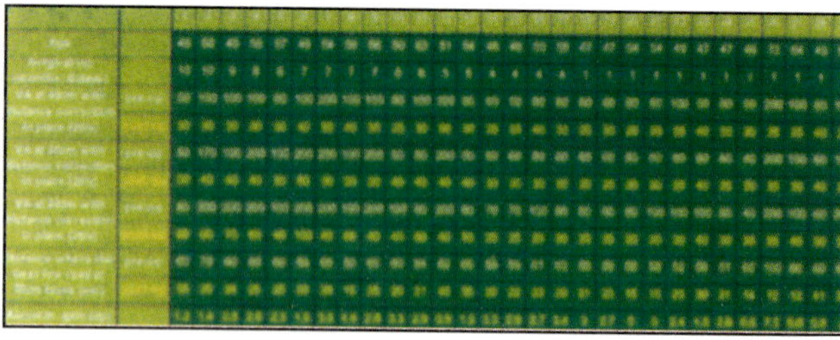

Fig. 13.14: Surgical reversal of presbyopia (SRP) accommodation results (Courtesy: Jean Pierre Maistre)

This study of 29 patients documents improved accommodation in all patients. Average near visual acuity improved by 4.8 lines. These patients had an average increase of 3.02 diopters of accommodation.

Lothringer's series of seven eyes, seven patients, aged 48 to 62 years, mean 153.3 years experienced a net dioptric increase in near point accommodation (NPA) of 3.13 diopters. This resulted in a net Snellen increase in near VA of six lines.

In these three studies, all patients experienced an increase in near point of accommodation. There was no loss of lines of best-corrected visual acuity (BCVA). There appeared to be no effect of the procedure on the distance refractive state.

Most interesting revelation to both the investigators and patients was the inordinate and unexpected increase in accommodation of the fellow eye in all cases (Fig. 13.15). This increase approached 20 to 50 percent of the increase measured when the surgery was performed on the dominant eye. The mechanism of these phenomena is not currently understood.

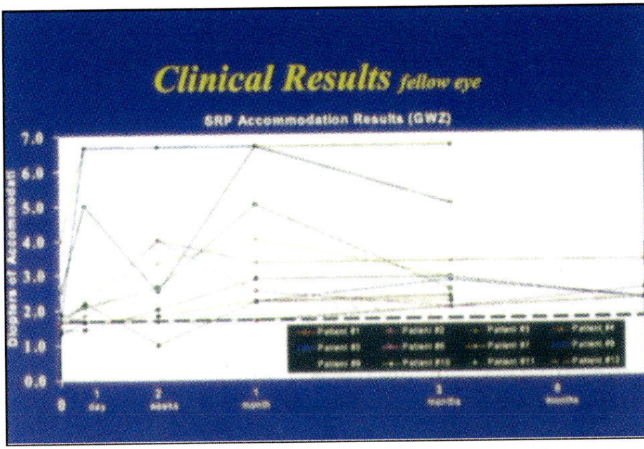

Fig. 13.15: Surgical reversal of presbyopia (SRP) accommodation results fellow eye (Courtesy: Gene W Zdenek)

Notice the effect in the fellow eye resembling the operative eye, but much less. The horizontal dashed line represents the average preoperative baseline accommodation (Fig. 13.16). Similar findings were documented in Maistre and Lothringer's data.

Typical appearance of a patient one month postoperatively. Note that the SEB segments are not visible in normal gaze. Under magnification, the inferiorly placed transparent SEB segments can often be observed while the patient looks in the superior gaze (Fig. 13.17).

Under high magnification, a typical SEB segment. Note the normal appearance of the conjunctiva overlying the segment. In the upper portion of this photograph, a remnant of a 10-0 nylon knot is present.

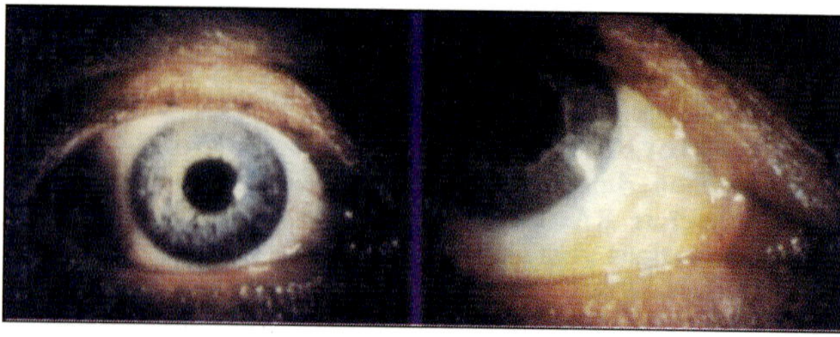

Fig. 13.16: Postoperative photographs (Courtesy: Gene W Zdenek)

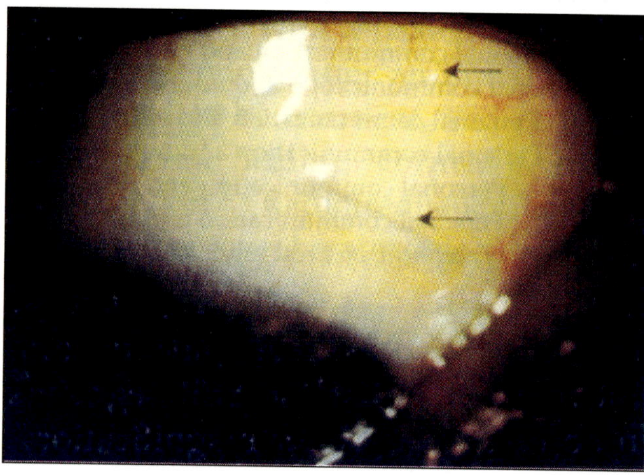

Fig. 13.17: Postoperative photograph (Courtesy: Gene W Zdenek)

Complications

To date, complications have been minor and rare. As in any surgical procedure, major complications could occur. SRP is a minimally invasive procedure. This, coupled with the fact that the investigative surgeons have been well trained, closely monitored and have adhered to the surgical protocol have resulted in the absence of any major complications. The following is the brief list of possible complications:

- Endophthalmitis (this has never occurred).
- Malignant glaucoma (this has never occurred with SEB segments) because this occurred with the full encircling bands, mannitol is still part of the current surgical protocol.
- Anterior segment ischemia (this has never occurred with the SEB segments). Important signs and symptoms to watch for are:
  1. Iris sector dilation (nonpharmacological)
  2. Descemet's folds—grayish in color
  3. Trace flare and cells
  4. Very low IOP
  5. Nausea.
- *SEB segment subluxation:* This is most commonly due to poor surgical technique or excessive rubbing of the eye by the patient in the early postoperative period.
- *SEB segment rotation:* This occurred in approximately 5 to 10 percent of the early designed SEB segments. This was the major reason for conjunctival erosion in the late postoperative period. The new SEB segment is wider, and should render this type of movement virtually impossible.
- *Conjunctival erosion:* When this occurs in the early postoperative period, the most common cause is

poor intraoperative conjunctival closure. This includes failure to recognize conjunctival tears or button holes.

- *Temporary keratoconjunctivitis:* The major cause of this is the temporary disruption of goblet cell function in the limbal region. In addition, malpositioning of the eyelid over the swollen conjunctiva and patients in an older age group contributes to this temporary condition.

The comfort level of this procedure for both the surgeon and patient lies in the fact that the SEB segments may be easily removed in the office at the slit-lamp under topical anesthetic in minutes.

SUMMARY

It is apparent that there are many flaws in the Helmholtz's theory of accommodation. This is best exemplified by the fact that researchers have been unable to duplicate a variable-focus single lens system similar to the human crystalline lens. Furthermore, Helmholtz's theory fails to have widespread applications to other scientific phenomena. In contrast, Schachar's theory not only has produced a variable-focus single element lens but also has widespread applications to many different scientific disciplines. For example, the mechanism by which the human crystalline lens deforms during accommodation is similar in mechanism to the counterintuitive shape changes of the earth's tides, the shape change of a drop of magnetic fluid within a magnetic field, and the similar but mysterious shape of many spiral galaxies that demonstrate central steepening and peripheral flattening.[16] What is truly amazing is the impact that Schachar's theory will have on the camera industry, defense industry (focusing on targets), optical computers and astronomy.

The visual correction revolution currently appears to be complete. Given the concept that presbyopia is a surgically correctable condition, the last major hurdle in refractive surgery has been overcome. While not everyone in the world needs glasses to see at distance, 100 percent of the population over the age of 40 will eventually need correction for presbyopia. The global impact of this immense population will be a driving force for the continued research and development of this procedure.

The anatomical modifications that scleral expansion bands produce in the ciliary muscle and trabecular meshwork may make this the procedure of choice for primary open-angle glaucoma. It is interesting to speculate the impact that SRP will have by allowing accommodation to continue during aging on the cataract prone crystalline lens.

REFERENCES

1. von Helmholtz H. Uber die akkommodation des auges. Albreckt von Graefe's Arch Ophthalmol 1885;1:89.

2. Fincham E. The mechanism of accommodation. Br J Ophthalmol 1937;8:1-9.
3. Schachar RA, Cudmore DP. The effect of gravity on the amplitude of accommodation. Ann Ophthalmol 1994;26: 65-70.
4. Koomen M, Tousey R, Scolnik R. The spherical aberration of the eye. J Opt Soc Am 1949;39:370-76.
5. Brown N. The change in shape and internal form of the lens of the eye on accommodation. Exp Eye Res 1973;15: 441-59.
6. Rafferty NS. Structure, function and pathology. In Maisel H (Ed): The Ocular Lens. New York: Marcel Dekker; 1985;2-5.
7. Atchison DA. Accommodation and presbyopia. Ophthalmic Physiol Opt 1995;15:255-72.
8. Kaufman PL, Rohen JW, Barany EH. Hyperopia and loss of accommodation following ciliary muscle disinsertion in the cynomolgus monkey—physiologic and scanning microscopic studies. Invest Ophthalmol Vis Sci 1979;18: 665-73.
9. Tamm S, Tamm E, Rohen JW. Age-related changes of the human ciliary muscle—a quantitative morphometric study. Mech Ageing Dev 1992;62:209-21.
10. Schachar RA. Cause and treatment of presbyopia with a method for increasing the amplitude of accommodation. Ann Ophthalmol 1992;24:445-52.
11. Schachar RA. Zonular function—a new hypothesis with clinical implications. Ann Ophthalmic 1994;26:36-38.
12. Schachar RA, Anderson DA. The mechanism of ciliary muscle function. Ann Ophthalmol 1995;27:126-32.
13. Schachar RA. Histology of the ciliary muscle-zonular connections. Ann Ophthalmol 1996;28:70-79.
14. Schachar RA, Cudmore DP, Black TD. A revolutionary variable focus lens. Ann Ophthalmol 1996;28:11-28.
15. Schachar RA, Cudmore DP, Black TD, et al. Paradoxical optical power increase of a deformable lens by equatorial stretching. Ann Ophthalmol 1998;30:10-18.

16. Schachar RA. Is Helmholtz's theory of accommodation correct? Ann Ophthalmol 1999;31:10-17.
17. Schachar RA. *In vivo* increase of the human lens equatorial diameter during accommodation. The American Physiological Society 1996;R670-76.
18. De la Garza Vi, Jose. Personal communication and notes.
19. Cross W. Personal communication and notes.
20. Yee R. Personal communication and notes.
21. Maistre JP. Personal communication and notes.
22. Zdenek G. Personal communication and notes.
23. Lothringer L. Personal communication and notes.
24. Schachar RA. Personal communication and notes.
25. Schachar RA. Treatment of Presbyopia and Other Eye Disorders, 1994, Slack.

CHAPTER 14

Solid State Lasers for Corneal Refractive Surgery

Matteo Piovella, Fabrizio I Camesasca, Barbara Kusa (Italy)

INTRODUCTION

Laser technology for refractive surgery advanced with unrelentless pace during the past 20 years. The introduction of concepts such as wavefront analysis and customized ablation required manifold developments dealing with an increased, outmost precision of treatment.

Solid-state lasers in ophthalmic surgery have meant increased energy efficiency, as well as reduced size and costs. Presently, a new generation of UV generating solid-state lasers is becoming available even for refractive surgery, including lasers such as the LaserSoft and the CustomVis.[1, 2]

KATANA, SOLID-STATE UV LASER FOR REFRACTIVE SURGERY SINCE 2003

A good example of solid-state laser for refractive surgery, LaserSoft, is a continuous wave diode-pumped all-solid-state UV laser for refractive surgery recently introduced by Katana Technologies GmbH. A solid-state is not an excimer laser, since the UV laser ablation radiation is generated by nonlinear frequency conversion of infrared laser light in a laser crystal. A sequential frequency conversion with nonlinear crystals shifts the wavelength of the laser radiation into the range of 208-210 nm. The resonator structure and the beam delivery ensure an emission of the laser radiation with a TEM_{00} transversal mode, as well as an emission of laser radiation with a true Gaussian beam. The continuous wave-diode pumping provides a very stable shot-to-shot UV output with impressive long-term stability.

A Gaussian beam means excellent UV light spot distribution on the cornea. In fact, differently from the usual excimer laser, the solid-state laser does not need beam-forming elements – i.e. mirrors - in the beam path. Thus, energy at the corneal surface – fluency – is very stable. The laser beam is highly collimated, providing an increased beam precision and the technical features adequate to a fast scanning. Furthermore, the ablation pattern utilized in LaserSoft ensures an extremely homogenous cornea surface due to the accurate overlap made possible by true Gaussian spots.

Differently from an excimer laser, in a solid-state laser there is no gas exchange and gas discharge involved, with the related instabilities in output radiation, due to the physical nature of the discharge process. The solid-state approach reduces the requirements for maintenance and costs, providing high stability and long lifetime.

This device generates a flying spot of 0.2 mm in diameter, operating at repetition rate of 1 kHz. Thanks to this high repetition rate, the energy per pulse is lower then in standard excimer treatments. Ablation has strongly reduced shock waves, and to no audible sound due to ablation or laser firing. The whole procedure takes place in a silent environment, much reassuring to the patient, without the risk of noise-induced abrupt motion.

To fully exploit the opportunities provided by custom ablation, a very fast laser like LaserSoft requires a fast eye-tracker. The LaserSoft eye-tracker has a latency of 1 ms and controls ablation centration at very high repetition rates. This very fast eye-tracker ensures a reliable, high repetition centration of ablation on the x-y axes as well as the ocular rotation.

All these features makes the solid-state laser an ideal device for accurate custom ablation (Figs 14.1 and 14.2).

The ablation profiles currently adopted by this laser are designed to preserve the strongly aspherical physiological corneal curvature, as well as to minimize the induced spherical aberration.

Different reflection losses and fluence values for different angles of incidence of the ablating laser radiation during surgery are also taken into account in the ablation algorithm.

CLINICAL EXPERIENCE

We hereafter illustrate our clinical experience with a solid-state laser. Patients were treated at two different centers: Messina (PRK) and Campobasso (LASIK), Italy. The results were gathered after one year and were analyzed with the software Datagraph, using graphs recommended by GO Waring III.[3, 4] After signing a specific informed consent, 37 eyes, were treated with LASIK and PRK procedures with LaserSoft ablation. Preoperative refractive data are reported in Table 14.1.

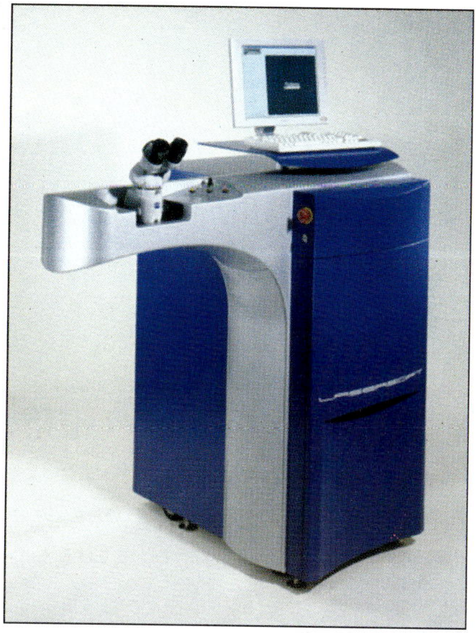

Fig. 14.1: LaserSoft solid-state laser

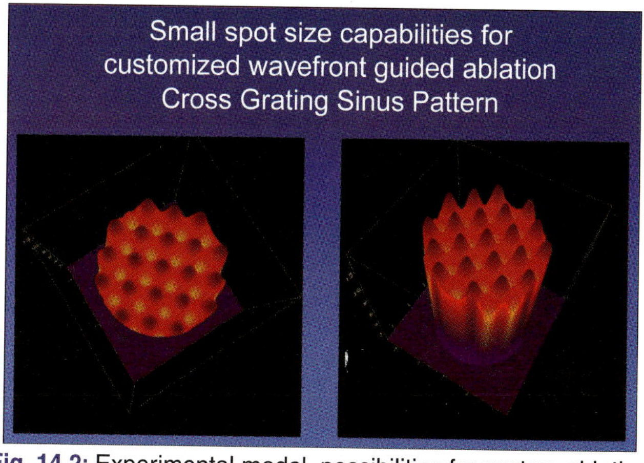

Fig. 14.2: Experimental model, possibilities for custom ablation offered by small spot size. Views of the attempted profile

Table 14.1: Preoperative vs one-month data, 37 eyes

	SE refractive defect (mean ± SD)	*Sphere (mean ± SD)*	*Cylinder (mean ± SD)*	*SE refractive defect, range*	*BSCVA*
Preoperative	–1.71 D ± 3.71 D	–1.46 D ± 3.32 D	–0.51 D ± 1.97 D	–8.00 D to +6.75 D	0.80 ± 0.23
One year	–0.03 D ± 0.13 D	–0.03 D ± 0.19 D	–0.01 D ± 0.19 D	–0.50 D to +0.25 D	0.83 ± 0.23

Preoperative BSCVA of all eyes was between 0.3 and 1.0. LASIK was performed with the Hansatome microkeratome, choosing a flap thickness of 180 micrometer. Treatment diameters ranged between 6 and 7 mm, and transition zones between 8 and 9 mm.

One-year results were well within the current standards provided by normal excimer lasers (Table 14.1). Figure 14.3 shows the scattergram of the attempted versus the achieved refractive change for each eye. Figure 14.4 shows the spherical equivalent refractive outcome with the corresponding numbers. At one year, 100 percent of the eyes were in the so called happiness zone of ± 1D, 94 percent were within ± 0.5 D, and 87 percent were within ± 0.25 D. Figure 14.5 shows stability of refraction. The mean achieved change of spherical equivalent with time is also given. Table 14.2 provides the refractive and BSCVA results at one year.

Efficacy consists of two components: component 1 is the spectacle corrected visual acuity at baseline (BSCVA); component 2 is the cumulative graph of uncorrected visual acuities after refractive surgery (UCVA). In our study, 45 percent of the eyes show a postoperative UCVA better then 20/20 from a cohort with 41 percent being preoperatively at 20/20 with best correction. The preoperative BSCVA of all eyes was between 1.0 and 0.3.

SOLID-STATE LASERS VS EXCIMER LASERS

Table 14.3 presents the differences between common excimer lasers and solid-state laser. Presently, solid-

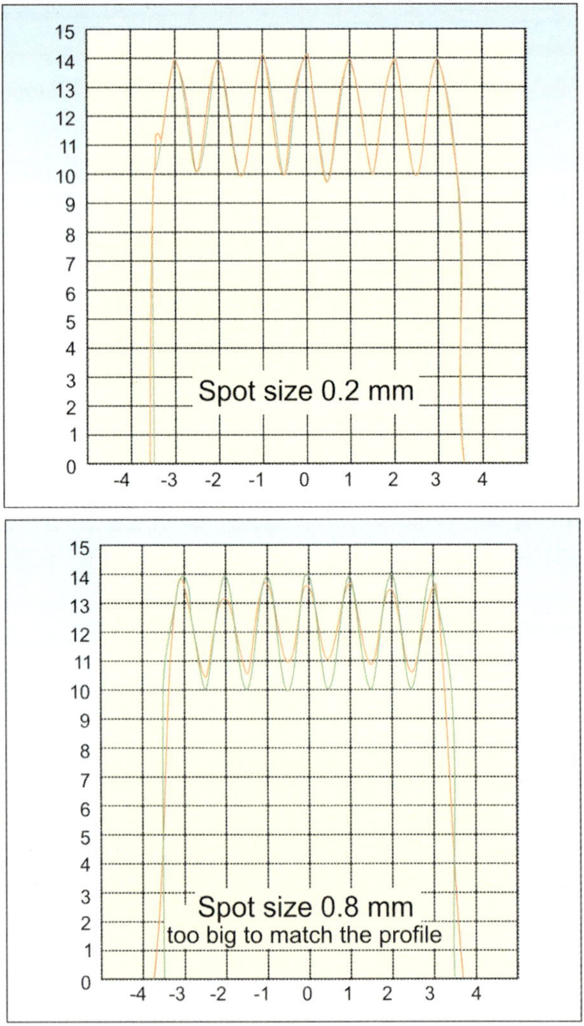

Fig. 14.3: Experimental model, small spot size and custom ablation. Views of the attempted profile with a 0.2 mm spot size solid-state laser vs. that of a 0.8 mm spot size

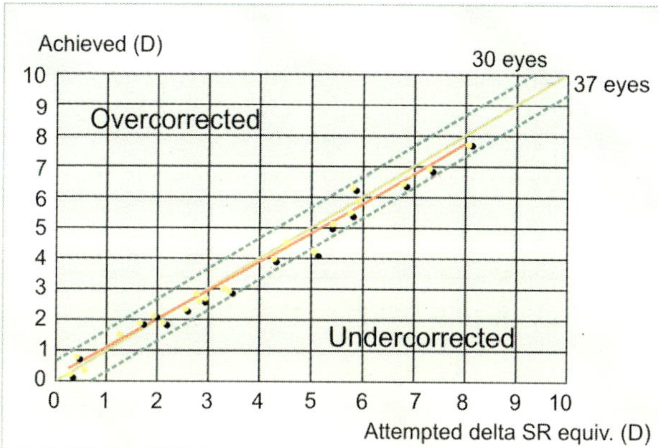

Fig. 14.4: Show the scattergram and therefore an impression of the spread of cases of the attempted versus the achieved refractive change for each eye for LASIK

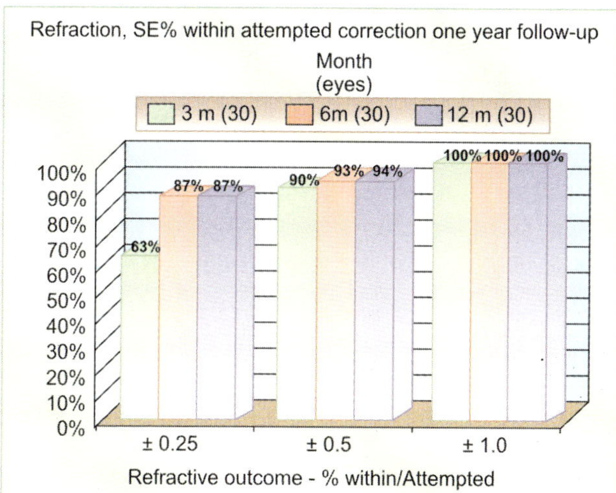

Fig. 14.5: Spherical equivalent refractive outcome at one year. Of all eyes, 100 percent are in the so-called happiness zone of ± 1D, 94 percent are within ± 0.5 D, and 87 percent are within ± 0.25 D

Table 14.2: Refractive and BSCVA results at one-year follow-up, 37 eyes

SE refractive defect, Attempted vs Obtained	*BSCVA Preoperative vs One-year*
–0.03 D ± 0.20 D	0.0 ± 0.2

state laser presents several significant examples of technical evolution in refractive surgery lasers. The solid-state laser features a tiny flying spot with a diameter of 0.2 mm and it operates at repetition rate of 1 kHz. Its very small spot size fits the present requirements for effective custom ablation.

The vast majority of excimer lasers commonly available on the market features a 1 mm flying spot, and they never have spots smaller than 0.65 mm, thus with a much wider spot ablation area than a solid-state laser (Fig. 14.6). There is a technical limit in decreasing the spot size of an excimer laser, as smaller spots would have a less homogeneous beam. Utilizing the usual excimer laser repetition rates, a 0.2 spot size would mean a very long treatment time, with the entire precision problem related to eye motion. To maintain ablation time within acceptable limits, and thanks to its technical features, the repetition rate of a solid-state laser is much higher in the solid-state than in excimer lasers.

The mirrors in a solid-state laser transmit the UV light without further elaborating it, unlike an excimer laser. This thanks to the true Gaussian profile of the beam.

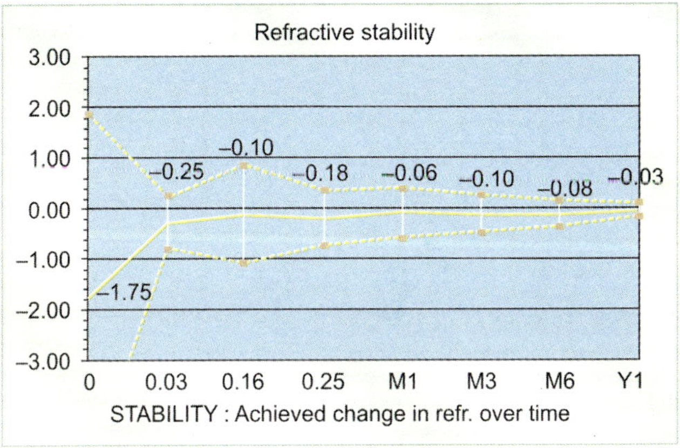

Fig. 14.6: Refractive stability of the study group, at one year

Table 14.3: Excimer vs solid-state lasers for refractive surgery

	Common excimer laser	*LaserSoft solid-state laser*
Spot size (mm)	0.8–1.0	0.2
Beam quality	Multimode (additional optics for clearing the excimer beam)	Single mode (Gaussian)
Repetition rate	50-500 Hz	1 kHz
Eye-tracker speed	Approximately 150 Hz	More than 1 kHz

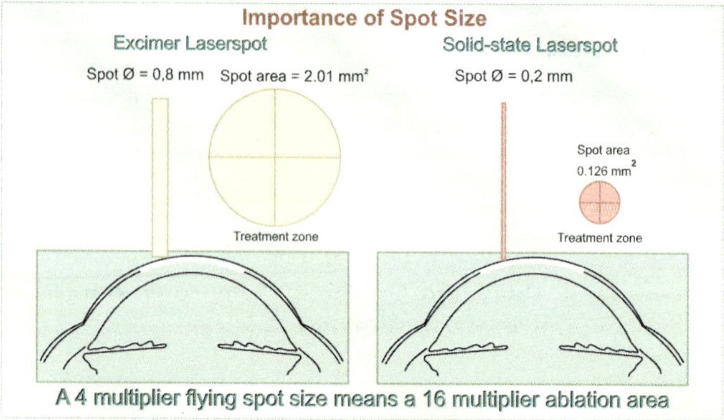

Fig. 14.7: Solid-state vs. excimer laser spot size

Solid-state lasers appear to be easier to use lasers for refractive surgery, requiring less maintenance.

The fast eye tracking ensures a reliable centration of ablation for x-y directions as well as the rotation of the eye at high repetition rates.

CONCLUSION

Solid-state lasers appear to be a promising solution for a refractive surgery, applying less energy to the cornea and using a small flying spot of 0.2 mm, thus with the theoretical potential of inducing less scarring.

LaserSoft and solid-state UV lasers in general appear as a safe, reliable, stable, more compact as well as less costly alternative to gas-operating excimer lasers for refractive surgery.

REFERENCES

1. Personal Communications, 2003 Meeting of the ISRS/AAO, November 14-15, 2003, Anaheim, CA. Syllabus 289.
2. Personal Communication, 2004 Meeting of the ISRS/AAO, October 22-23, 2004, New Orleans, LA. Syllabus 10.
3. Datagraph med (Medical Data Analysis Software) Ingenieurbüro Pieger, Germany.
4. Waring G. Standard Graphs for Reporting Refractive Surgery. J Refract Surg 2000;16:459.

CHAPTER 15

Presbyopic Multifocal LASIK (PML): A New Approach in Presbyopia Correction

Roberto Pinelli (Italy)

INTRODUCTION

In all refractive surgery, our goal has been to surgically correct the visual defects, i.e. myopia, hyperopia, astigmatism, and presbyopia. Correction of these defects is possible through corneal surgical procedures or lenticular surgery.

Of all the visual defects, presbyopia has been the most challenging to correct, partly because the mechanisms of accommodation and the causes of presbyopia are complex and not fully understood. Thus far, it has largely been managed through the use of progressively stronger spectacles, which gradually take over the near focus work of the crystalline lens. Presbyopia is also unique in that it is the only refractive error that is considered to be progressive in nature. Although our management and most of our experience seems to point to the progressive nature of presbyopia, in truth, we do not know for sure that it truly progresses. It may be that in our "prosthetic culture" we have merely become unnecessarily dependent on our glasses and contacts.

In any case, a surgical alternative to the correction of presbyopia is appealing because of the enormous pool of presbyopic patients with a desire for good uncorrected vision. Mild hyperopes and emmetropes who have never worn glasses are particularly uncomfortable with presbyopia and its associated inconveniences.

APPROACHES TO THE SURGICAL CORRECTION OF PRESBYOPIA

The mission of presbyopic surgery—as with all other refractive surgeries—should be to eliminate the symptoms of the refractive error, rather than to correct the anatomical defect itself. For this reason, I think an approach that provides pseudoaccommodation is natural and appropriate. If we can provide patients with good functional vision at multiple distances, it is not necessary to restore true accommodative function in the form of a dynamically adjusting optical power of the eye.

There are several potential sites for correction of presbyopia. The cornea is probably the most common target, as it is the area refractive surgeons are most comfortable operating on. Theoretically, the anterior chamber provides another site for the correction of presbyopia, but this is as yet theoretical and would likely prove extremely difficult in reality. The human crystalline lens can be replaced with a multifocal or accommodative intraocular lens, of which many different styles are now underdevelopment and coming to market. Finally, a number of scleral implant or ciliary muscle surgical procedures have been developed. This approach, however, is complicated, largely untested, and seems "more surgical" than is necessary.

As a familiar corneal procedure, LASIK has been the most popular and easiest surgical approach. In addition to the surgeon comfort level with the procedure, patients in the presbyopic baby boomer generation are also familiar with and accepting of the procedure. In addition, LASIK can be performed bilaterally on the same day, is relatively quick and painless, and has proven to be quite safe.

Even with LASIK, we have several options for addressing presbyopia. Most conventionally, we have taken a monofocal approach with surgically-induced monovision, but bifocal and multifocal approaches are increasing. LASIK is ideal for presbyopia because of the absence of haze and its associated refractive complications, the absence of regression, and the presence of a regular and, hopefully, thin flap that can protect the multifocality created in the stroma.

In designing a multifocal LASIK procedure, we must take advantage of some of the lessons learned from current and past procedures. Some myopes treated with radial keratotomy have retained good near and distance vision well into the presbyopic age range. Why is that? Similarly, some hyperopic LASIK patients also have retained their pseudoaccommodative function well into their older years. Again, why would that be? The secret lies in the asphericity of the cornea. A prolate cornea seems to have the capability to focus both far and near better than an oblate cornea. We have seen that again recently with conductive keratoplasty, which I perform and have been involved in studying in Italy. CK is an excellent technique for correcting hyperopia and restoring near vision. It appears to provide some degree of multifocality because eyes corrected for near visual acuity with CK typically have much better distance visual acuity than would be expected. This may be due to the prolateness of the post-CK cornea. In any case, the "blended vision" of CK permits the presbyopic patient to read by treating just the nondominant eye.

In the past three years, my purpose has been to create a truly multifocal corneal procedure that can be performed bilaterally if necessary, and that will work for any eye, regardless of preoperative refractive error. Intuitively, we know that many zones should do a better job of mimicking natural vision than just two zones, but obtaining a gradual but effective multifocality is nonetheless challenging. The ultimate presbyopic LASIK procedure must also be easy to perform, with standardized nomograms that any surgeon can use as a basis for successful surgery.

THE PML™ PROCEDURE

With the above goals in mind, I developed and have been investigating at ILMO a patented procedure which we call PML™ (Presbyopic Multifocal LASIK). This procedure can be performed on presbyopic myopes, hyperopes, astigmats, and emmetropes. Multifocality on the cornea is created using a multi-step treatment in which several independently calculated ablations are performed at various optical

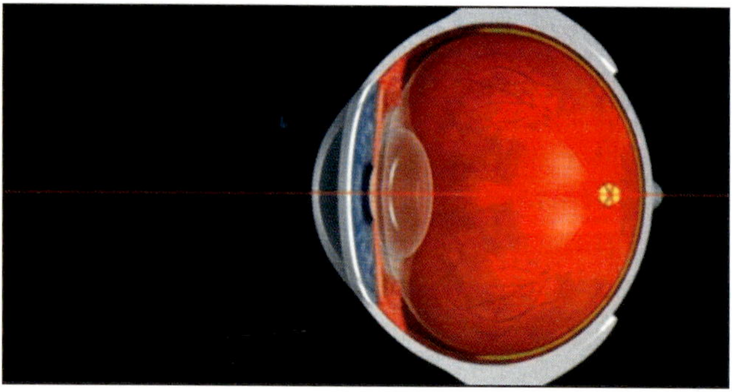

Fig. 15.1: Central area of the cornea: Focus on the retina

zones. Depending on the patient's refractive error, there may be anywhere from three to eight different concentric zones. In all cases, the goal is to treat the central cornea for distance vision, with a multifocal peripheral cornea that is able to provide functional near vision. Some other multifocal LASIK procedures take the opposite approach, with the near correction in the center. However, the central cornea provides an excellent site for distance vision because it is relatively aberration-free, while peripheral aberrations may actually be useful for near focusing.

In this multi-step process, we first treat astigmatism in the classic manner, as if we were doing a purely astigmatic laser correction. Next we treat the distance defect in a zone on the central cornea. Then, we treat the near defect in a larger optical zone. Finally, other zones may be created to ensure that the overall power of the cornea is emmetropic, even though there are varying powers in the different optical zones. It is a procedure that is highly customizable for each patient's optical needs.

I began doing this procedure in 2002, starting cautiously by treating 10 patients in only their non-dominant eyes. One year postoperatively, five of these patients were happy with their outcomes; the other five required retreatment. These unilateral patients experienced some of the benefits and problems of monovision. I became convinced that a bilateral approach would be more effective, and began to adjust and refine the nomograms towards this end.

For our first bilateral study cohort, we treated 100 eyes of 50 patients with. Our studies so far have been performed with the Technolas 217 Z (Bausch and Lomb) and the Lasitome microkeratome (Gebauer). However, the procedure is technology-independent

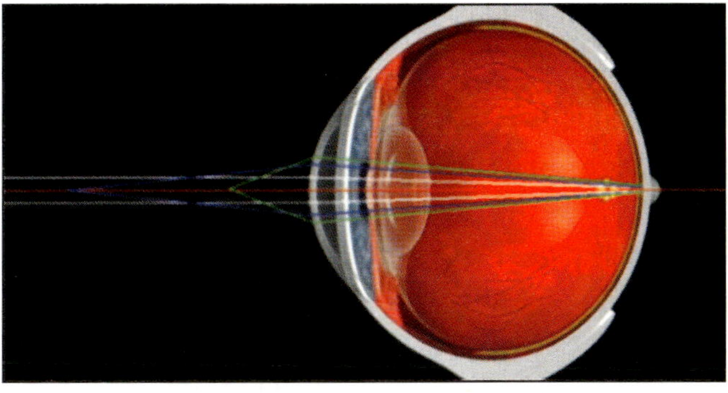

Fig. 15.2: Multifocality permits to focus both far and near objects on macula (pseudoaccommodation)

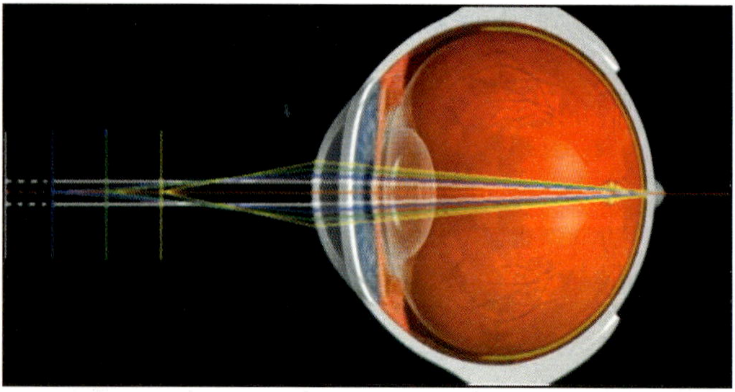

Fig. 15.3: Effects of a completely multifocal cornea

and was designed to work with any keratome and laser combination.

RESULTS

All 50 patients were seeing at least 20/25 for distance and at least J3 for near. Eighty percent had bilateral uncorrected vision of 20/20 or better for distance and J2 or better for near. Another 10 percent were 20/25 and J2, while the remaining 10 percent were 20/25 and J3. Patient satisfaction levels have been very high, and there have been no retreatments thus far. Typically, patients experience a myopic shift during the first month postoperatively, then stabilize at plano.

A few cases illustrate well the potential of this procedure. The first example is a 50-year-old female who was a –6.0 D myope with a +1.5 D add for reading. We treated the cornea in six different zones: a –1.5 D

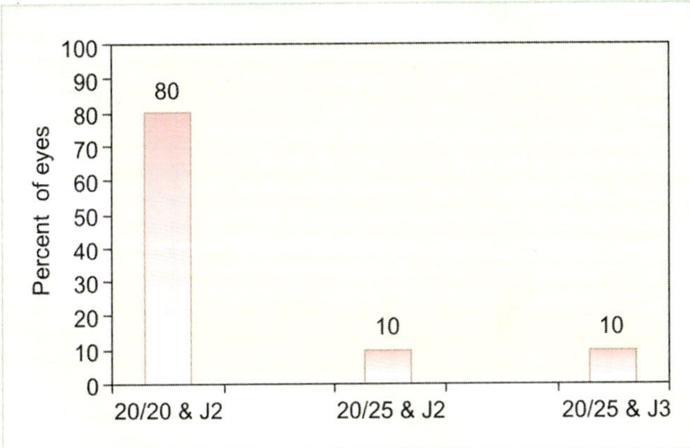

Fig. 15.4: 50 patients' eyes postoperative results

correction in each of the following optical zones: 4.8, 5.2, 5.4, 5.6, and 6.0 mm; and a +2.00 D correction at the 6.5 mm optical zone. Six months postoperative her uncorrected vision is 20/20 and J2 in both eyes.

The second case is a 54-year-old patient who was plano in both eyes preoperatively but using a +1.5 D add for near vision. We performed two treatment rings for near vision, each +0.75 D, at the 6.0 and 6.5 mm optical zones. In addition, I did three treatment rings for distance vision, ablating a –0.50 D spherical correction at the 5.0, 5.2, and 5.4 mm optical zones. After a myopic reaction initially, the eyes are now emmetropic, and six months postoperative, this patient's uncorrected visual acuity is 20/20 and J2 in both eyes. Ultimately, my goal is to be able to correct emmetropes like this as soon as they start experiencing presbyopic symptoms at age 45 or 50.

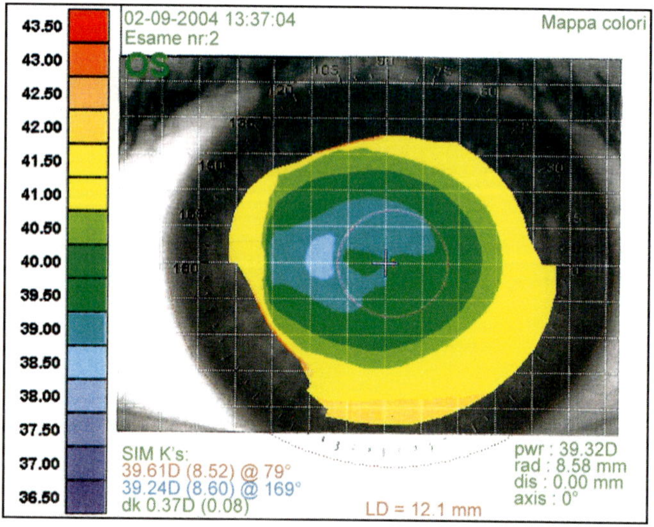

Fig. 15.5: A prolate cornea after PML™ case # 1

PEARLS AND LESSONS LEARNED

We have found that it is better to overcorrect hyperopia and to undercorrect myopia, and that astigmatism must be fully corrected for a satisfactory outcome. In some cases (hyperopes and emmetropes), the cornea becomes more prolate; in other cases (primarily myopes) it actually becomes more oblate. Pupil size is not an important factor in determining outcomes from this procedure. We have not had to manage patients with especially large pupils any differently than we would with a monofocal LASIK procedure.

The PML™ technique uses the same or less tissue as other laser vision correction procedures, so although

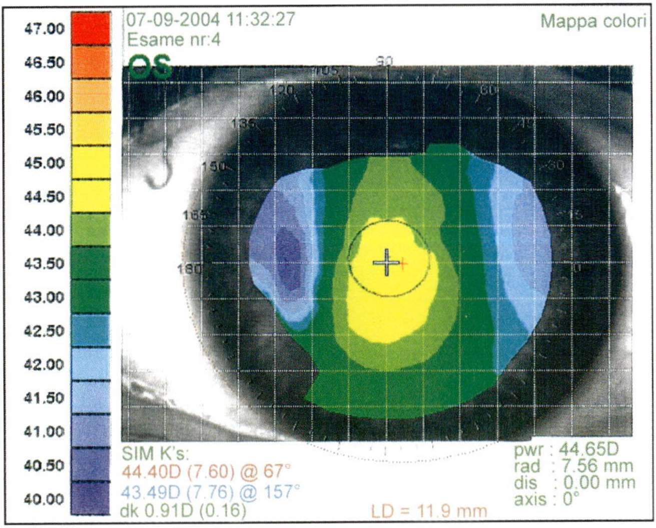

Fig. 15.6: An oblate cornea after PML™ case # 2

pachymetry is important, it is no more a factor than in monofocal LASIK. Keratometry is very important, as it is essential to keep the pre- and postoperative K values constant.

Patients must be willing to participate in training their eyes to learn how to see at near with the multifocal correction. Our patients are instructed not to use reading glasses after the procedure at all and to do visual exercises (for which we provide instruction) in order to maintain the eye's focusing power with age.

In our experience so far, is a very successful procedure that has been well-accepted by patients and is in high demand at our center. Currently, about 30 percent of our patients are PML™ candidates. The procedure and the excellent results experienced by patients have enhanced the reputation of our center and generated many referrals. Ongoing research is required to determine whether and when regression might occur.

CHAPTER 16

VisioDynamics Theory: A Biomechanical Application for the Aging Eye and Laser ACE™ Natural Vision Restoration

AnnMarie Hipsley (USA)
Dimitrii Dementiev (Italy)

INTRODUCTION

VisioDynamics: Biomechanical Model for the Aging Ocular Organ

The defining concept of VisioDynamic Theory is that *presbyopia is not a refractive error or simply the loss in the ability to focus on near objects, rather it is an Aging Disease* whereas the age-related consequences on connective tissue as they occur throughout the body produce significant but reversible impact on biomechanical efficiency of ocular function which includes visual function, ocular biotransport, and ocular metabolic efficiency among other ocular organ functions.[1] The limiting factors for eye function throughout development and during aging can be broken down into *three* basic categories:

- Structural/mechanical
- Physiological
- Extracellular and intracellular.

Connective tissues (CT) can change their strength depending on the forces applied to them. Without force acting on them, the chemical structures and property of the tissues change, and therefore the fibers and mechanical properties of the tissue change. In muscle tissue this is called atrophy; in other supporting CT this is called hysteresis.[2] The SAID (Specific Adaptation to Imposed Demands) principle applies here, whereas the internal design of CT works as a feedback loop which is responsive to force, mass and gravity.[3] The opposite can happen if a CT begins to receive a persistent stress. If you do something to stress the CT, it will gradually add new CT at the point of stress, this is called hypertrophy.

The *internal design of* CT also responds to organismal experience such as environmental stress, biological stress, chemical stress which can manifest itself into various disease processes or traumas if the cycle is not broken. CT remodels itself in order to accommodate the new stress.[4] Chronic stress which exceeds the threshold of tissue healing can produce a low-grade chronic inflammatory process which triggers a cycle of cell damage ultimately resulting in cell death and or irreversible tissue changes which affect homeostatic equilibrium—this is 'aging'.[5] Despite the normal loss of elastin, collagen and dehydration of tissue, tissue morphology is limited by genetic predisposition, cultural (race) and environmental (altitude/sunlight) impact and inherent structural characteristics of health.[6] In the VisioDynamic Theory, the loss of accommodation in presbyopia is due to age-related changes of the eye which affect its normal biomechanical and therefore physiological function.[7] Biomechanical dysfunction leads to increased mechanical load, shear stress and consequential tissue strain. Tissue strain and deformation has effects on micro tissue layer interactions, collagenous integral structure/remodeling and ultimately extracellular matrix chemical and nutrient balance and efficiency.[8] Tissue properties and

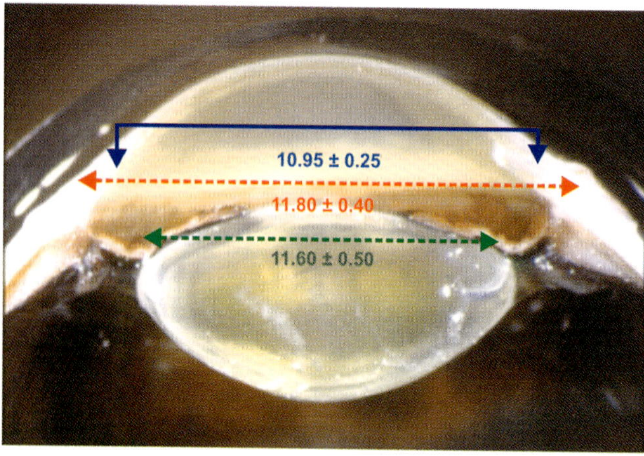

Fig. 16.1: Biomechanical relationship of ocular structures *in vivo:* White-to-white; Anterior chamber diameter, Ciliary sulcus diameter

architecture are critical considerations when determining the impact of the pathophysiology of age-related changes (Fig. 16.1).[9] The cornea is responsible for two-thirds of the eye's total focusing power, while the crystalline lens accounts for the remaining one-third. The focusing power of the cornea is fixed, whereas focusing power of lens complex is not fixed and depends largely on the mechanical efficiency of accommodation mechanism which is dependent upon the biomechanical relationships of the structures of the eye. Therefore, any surgical solution implemented for an aging ocular organ would be enhanced by restoring biomechanical balance in the structures included in the *Kinematic chain* of the *Oculociliary complex*.

BIOMECHANICAL IMPACT OF AGE-RELATED CHANGES IN OCULAR TISSUE

Biomechanical Dysfunction Hypothesis

The *biomechanical dysfunction hypothesis* postulates that there is a highly-structured inter-relationship in terms of the homeostatic stimuli which are shared in common by different ocular tissues as suggested by the close anatomic and functional relationship which they have evolved from.[1] Biomechanical efficiency relies on: **or ME = W × 100/E – e** *where E is the gross energy output, e is the resting metabolic rate, and W is the external work performed.* Optimal positive work or mechanical efficiency of ocular organ function occurs when this equation is balanced.[10] Every joint has a particular biomechanical arrangement with its associated musculature which is crucial to structure composition and form against gravity (posture) and the coordination of the neuromuscular units of the joint to produce the resultant force necessary to perform movement (function).[11] Restoring normal biomechanical relationships to the aging oculus facilitates the ocular structures to work with gravity in the most efficient way: The *oculociliary joint* is "postured" into optimum position to allow for the maximum potential kinetic energy to perform positive work or anterior acceleration and posterior deceleration of the lens for maximum range of dynamic visual tasks.[12] Biomechanical balance and specificity allows for efficient ocular movement, whereas, biomechanical dysfunction demands compensatory movements (due to over- or inappropriate loading) which will be 'patterned' and eventually interfere with performance. The accommodative mechanism is system of levers, and static contractions are responsible for the discrete adjustments to hold these levers in optimal alignment. The 'posture' of the lens during disaccommodation is an important baseline for determining the functional capacity of the accommodative mechanism.[13] By gaining increasing control over these processes, biomechanical proficiency increases. The LaserACE™ procedure or (Laser Anterior Ciliary Excision) was developed based on the fundamentals of biomechanics, neurophysiology, and kinesiology of the aging eye organ.[14] This procedure effectively and naturally restores the biomechanical inter-relationships of the intraocular structures providing biomechanical efficiency and alleviating biomechanical dysfunction by decreasing anterior global scleral compression load and subsequent subliminal tissue stress, strain and deformation.[15,16]

Scleral Compression Hypothesis

The sclera undergoes a gradual "sclerosclerosis" with age which represents the normal and gradual irreversible changes which occur in all connective tissues as we aged.[17] In addition, increased ocular rigidity has been linearly correlated with age.[18] This

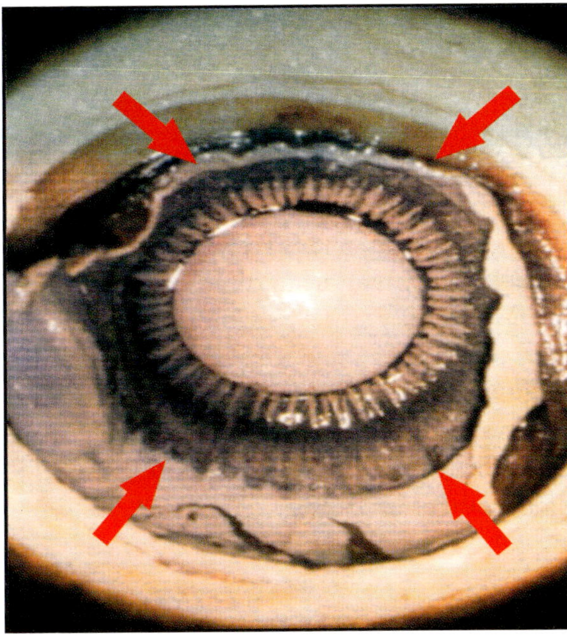

Fig. 16.2: Scleral load vectors on underlying structures

sclerotic process imposes staggeringly significant load, stress and strain upon underlying and related ocular and intraocular structures[19,20] (Fig. 16.2). Every tissue inter-related with the sclera, therefore, will respond according to the SAID principle or otherwise respond by Specific Adaptation to Imposed Demands. CT of the ocular organ adapts to stress by compensation, substitution, or overload.[21]

Subsequently, all structures within the ocular organ sustain a 'gradual accumulation of microtrauma' over time. *Aging is a cyclical low-grade inflammatory process ultimately resulting in irreversible changes in tissue. Unless the cycle is broken, cell death, organ death, system death and eventually organismal death occurs.* Age-related changes in connective tissue of sclera include changes in collagen composition of GAGs (glycosaminoglycans), thickness, rigidity, tissue architecture (angle recession and changed biomechanical relationships), and changes homeostatic response.[22-24] Until now, the complex interaction of the sclera and recognition of its huge impact on the internal processing and diffusive mechanism in the eye organ has been considerably overlooked.[25] Age-related changes in the sclera are directly relative, indirectly relative or concomitantly relative to the impairment of the functional performance of the entire eye organ.[26] The majority of the inner anatomical and physiological areas of eye organ function lie beneath 5/6 of the outer tunic or the sclera which makes this structure a critical tissue consideration in terms of age-related changes in CT and its impact on biomechanical function of the eye organ.[27,28] One of the most critical zones is in the area of the limbus at the corneoscleral envelope (Fig. 16.3).[29] A primary limiting factor in the ability to respond to near stimulus through the accommodative mechanism is the loss of mobility of the sclera. The magnitude of the response to near stimulus is also limited by the degree of "sclerosclerosis" or age-related fibrosis of the sclera. Muscular imbalance, which develops from biomechanical dysfunction can ultimately involve the whole

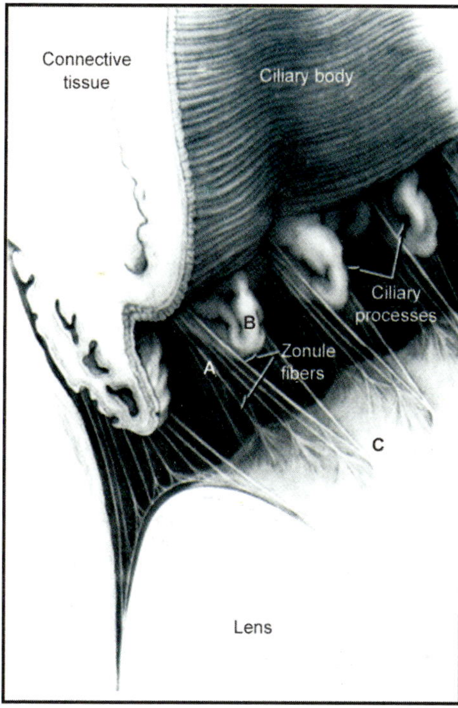

Fig. 16.3: Physiology of the limbal structures underlying sclera at corneoscleral envelope

ocular organ and even body function. All of these underlying structures are impacted by the progressive scleral load either directly or indirectly creating such dysfunction as ONH atrophy, choroid dysfunction/ vascular insufficiency, decreased uveal-aqueous outflow, increased IOP, biomechanical dysfunction of EOM, and ultimately gross disturbances in ICM and ECM metabolic transport. ECM and metabolic transport.[30-32]

In vivo, CT *mobility* is important for the normal maintenance and turnover of PG (proteoglycan) in healthy tissue. Conversely, tissue *immobilization* or disuse results in atrophy because of a loss of PG from the matrix.[33] However, it is also noted in research that this PG loss following immobilization is *reversible* if normal tissue conditions and more importantly when *mobility* is restored.[34] Age-related effects of connective tissue can have enormous impact specific to overlying sclera shell thickness. "Structure = Function" is at the crux of the VisioDynamic model and is instrumental in the hypothesis and application of the LaserACE™ procedure which is based on restoring the biomechanical relationships of the ocular tunic in critical zones of physiological importance.[35] A state of equilibrium is reached and the internal stress balances the applied load (Fig. 16.4). The principal goal of LaserACE™ procedure is to decrease the overall applied load stress by decompression of sclerotic CT load, to restore mobility, to rejuvenate physiological functions in the anterior globe and further retard tissue strain and deformation rates in the aging eye. The fundamental objective is to restore essential biomechanical components which are affected by age-related pathology and promote longevity of the ocular organ.

Principle: Specific Adaptation to Imposed Demands (SAID)

Force and *friction* play a large role in ocular functional capacity. Leonardo da Vinci has the credit to be the first

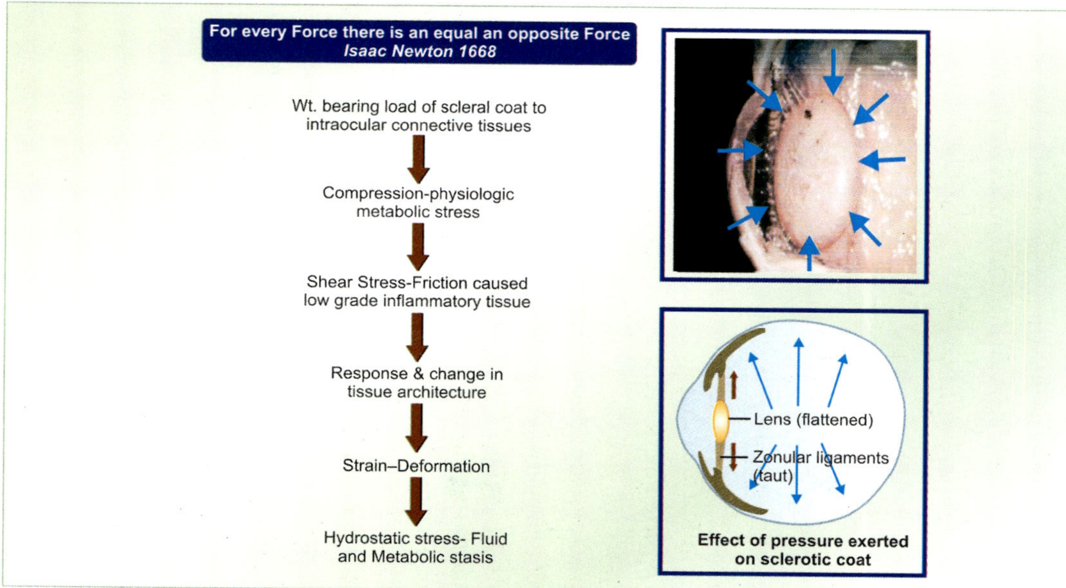

Fig. 16.4: Scleral coat load creates an internal stress response of elevated IOP to achieve equilibrium

who made quantitative studies on the problem of friction. Leonardo defined a friction coefficient as the ratio of the friction divided by the mass of the slider. Experimentally, he found a universal friction coefficient of 0.25 independent of the material. Ocular tissues like other biological tissues like to live in a homeostatic stress/strain range. Therefore, force (mass × acceleration) and friction play a critical role in the ability for aging ocular tissue to function efficiently. Values of stress/strain outside of this range will lead to adaptation and changes in the tissue structure.[36] The *SAID principle* for ocular aging states that: *Age-related changes which occur in connective tissue increase both the static and dynamic coefficient of friction. Constant and gradual increased force and mass of the scleral load on underlying ocular tissues elicits equal and opposite force requirements resulting in intraocular physiological overload. Increased friction and load stress across tissue layers further elicits a cycle of repetitive low-grade inflammatory tissue responses, changes in tissue architecture, connective tissue deformation, and biomechanical dysfunction Specific to Imposed Demands which overall decrease biomechanical efficiency of ocular organ function.* Therefore, there is a constant linear deceleration of intraocular physiological processes concomitant with increased moment of inertia produced by progressive age-related scleral force (load) and friction (stress-strain).

BIOMECHANICAL SOLUTIONS FOR THE AGING OCULAR ORGAN

History of Biomechanical Surgical Solutions

During the mid 1970s in Russia, Fyodorov began treating myopia (near sightedness) in patients using radial or spoke cuts through the cornea to biomechanically flatten its shape.[37] The biomechanics of the RK surgery evolved further to the limbal region and to the sclera after surgeons noticed unanticipated impact on other visual functions (Fig. 16.5).

Scleral ablation was first hypothesized as a treatment for presbyopia shortly after RK was brought to the United States (Fig. 16.6). Surgeons (particularly a group led by Spencer Thornton, MD) began to notice

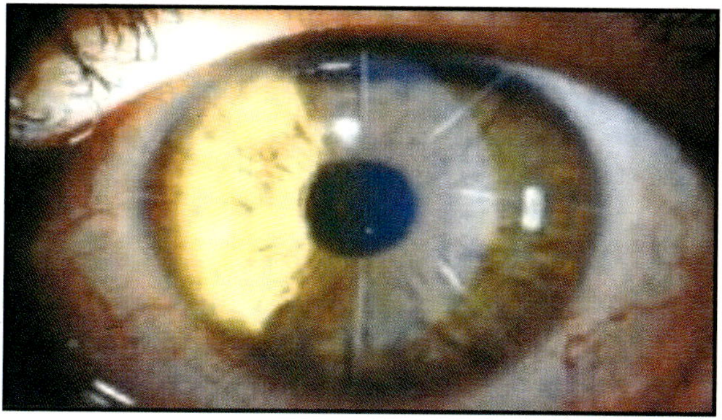

Fig. 16.5: Early biomechanical applications in the cornea (RK)

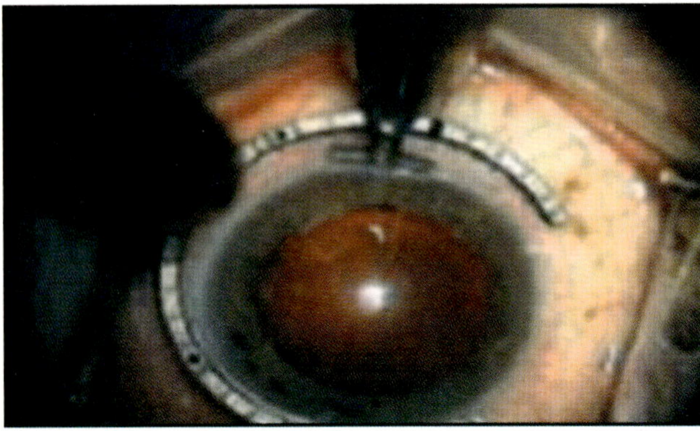

Fig. 16.6: Thornton developed one of the first presbyopic specific procedure using scleral incisions: Anterior ciliary sclerotomy (ACS)

that some of their patients were not developing presbyopia as expected. It appeared that this was by product of RK surgery when the radial incision went through the limbus.

Dr Thornton organized a group of leading RK surgeons worldwide to perform scleral incisions and test this theory. While the procedure held promise, the results were less dramatic mainly due to regression as the incisional sites healed. Only a small increase in the amplitude of accommodation was observed and .5 D of myopic shift was also recorded.[38] This procedure later evolved to be combined with silicone plugs having a more impressive and lasting effect. "ACS" is currently in clinical trials.

Schachar hypothesized a new model of accommodation controversial to the Helmholtz theory and performed scleral implants over the ciliary body in order to achieve an increase in accommodative power. (Scleral Expansion Bands "SEB"). He hypothesized that the primary element in achieving the accommodative effect was the increase in the working distance for the ciliary muscle complex.[39]

JT Lin hypothesized that the effect of scleral incisions was not permanent due to the rapid healing response of the body and utilized an Er:YAG laser to make the incisions. Under this technique, LPC or LAPR, near full thickness ablations of the sclera are made in parallel radial orientation in the four quadrants resulting in an axial length change and anterior globe expansion.[40]

Hipsley introduced VisioDynamic Theory in 2003 based on the effects caused by the age-related changes of CT on the inner structures of critical physiological functional importance and countered that increasing scleral diameter across the globe was not ideal and in fact could superimpose even more biomechanical imbalance and possible instability to an already homeostatically challenged structure.[41] LaserACE™ procedure was developed based upon these fundamental principles of age-related changes on connective tissues and their progress load, stress/strain on subliminal tissues of the eye and imposing biomechanical dysfunction and its effects on ocular function.

LaserACE™ Biomechanical Surgical Solution

Unlike the expansion procedures, LaserACE™ is distinctly different in that it is a *decompression* procedure

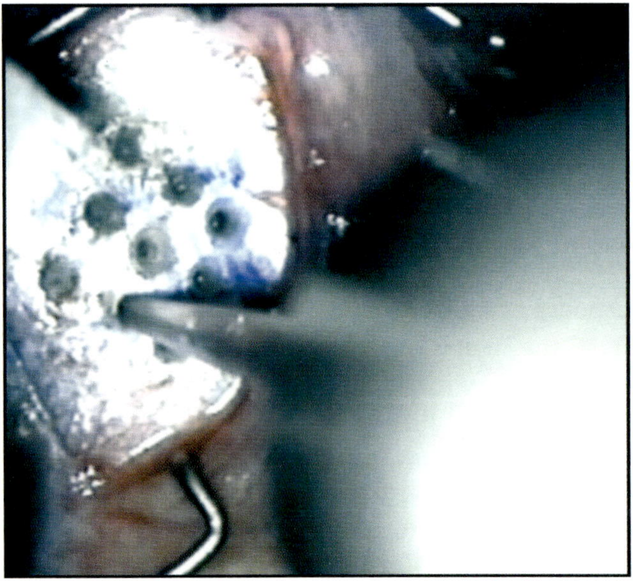

Fig. 16.7: LaserACE^{TM} "NeoPore" matrix decompressing fibrotic scleral mass and restoring physiological function

which emphasizes volumetric excisions in a CT matrix over critical segmental zones of fibrotic sclera in addition to creating a mechanical diaphragm pump in aponeurotic layers of the eye to rejuvenate aqueous outflow and alleviate stress from sensory receptors (Fig. 16.7). Restoration of the Biomechanics of Accommodation with LaserACE^{TM} or Laser Anterior Ciliary Excision is performed utilizing the patented VisioLite ophthalmic laser system with optical probe (Fig. 16.12A).

- Since nothing can be done about lenticular hardening on must aim to increase the biomechanical efficiency of oculociliary joint complex.

- Restoration of biomechanical balance requires alleviating restrictions and maximizing intraocular structural functional performance without imposing new biomechanical challenges to the oculus.
- Resultant effects of LaserACE™ allow for a new static oculociliary joint complex resting posture which maximizes the kinetic potential of the neuromuscular system.
- Resultant effects of decompression rejuvenate ocular biotransport mechanisms both indirectly and dynamically.

To distinguish LaserACE™ from scleral expansion procedures: Scleral expansion procedures have been proposed by Thornton ACS (Anterior Ciliary Sclerotomy), Fukusaku, Schachar (Scleral Expansion Bands), and LAPR procedure. Scleral expansion procedures are primarily based on the "Lens Crowding Theory" and strive to achieve improvement of the working distance of the ciliary complex or the circumlental space by inducing a 'pseudomyopic' eye shape with the polar axis longer than the equatorial diameter. Scleral implants are inserted into the superficial tunnels, causing a slight lift or 'myopic roof' in the sclera designed to reduce the crowding of the underlying muscles surrounding the crystalline lens. Alternatively, a radial ablation technique is used to create full thickness expansion of the anterior globe of the sclera producing enough substantial relaxing of the scleral tissue in the anterior globe to effectively change the stability of the anterior globe significantly enough to produce a myopic shift and axial length change. All of the expansion procedures have significant effects on eye shape of the anterior globe as a primary mechanism of action. LaserACE™ is *theoretically* different from the expansion procedures regarding the etiology of loss of ocular function as well as the mechanism and principles of restoration of ocular function. LaserACE™ procedure is based on the VisioDynamic Theory and scleral compression, biomechanical dysfunction, homeostatic, and neuromuscular hypotheses.[1] In this model, the etiology of the loss of accommodation in presbyopia is principally related to the effects of age-related changes of the eye which impact its normal biomechanical functions.[42] Scleral compression ultimately precipitates ocular biomechanical dysfunction leading to increased mechanical load, shear stress and consequential tissue strain.[43] Tissue strain and deformation has effects on micro tissue layer interactions, collagenous integral structure/remodeling and ultimately neuromuscular, physiological and extracellular matrix chemical and nutrient balance and efficiency. LaserACE™ surgical application is fundamentally different from these procedures in that there is no objective for scleral expansion or induced myopia, rather there is a zonal decompression of the connective tissue restriction which eliminates the compression or impingement of subliminal connective tissue, fascal tissue, and biophysiological structures of the eye organ (Fig. 16.8).

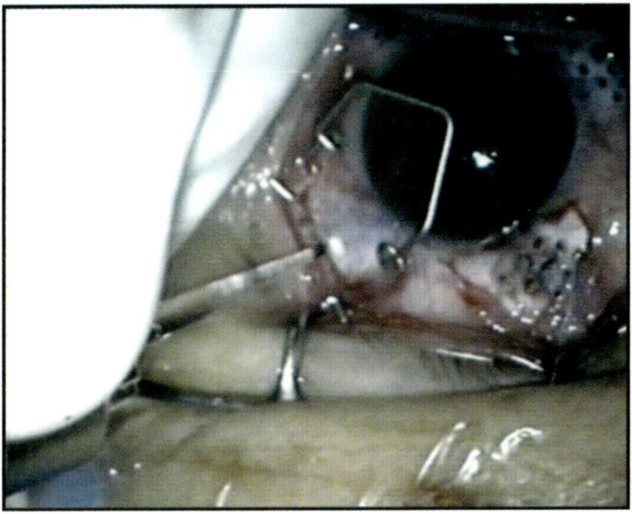

Fig. 16.8: LaserACE™ zonal decompression decreases vertical load and creates no expansion

LaserACE™ Strategic Critical Zones of Restoration

LaserACE™ nomogram is based on mathematical calculations in anterior globe sphere specific to three critical zones (Figs 16.9 and 16.10). The key element in the effectiveness of the procedure lies in the ability to decompress the anterior globe with specificity to the key physiological and biomechanical areas of function. It is also critical to create the micro "NeoPores" with respect to the geometry of the sphere and the relative change in scleral thickness, CT characteristics, and rigidity across the globe (Fig. 16.9). The cylindrical

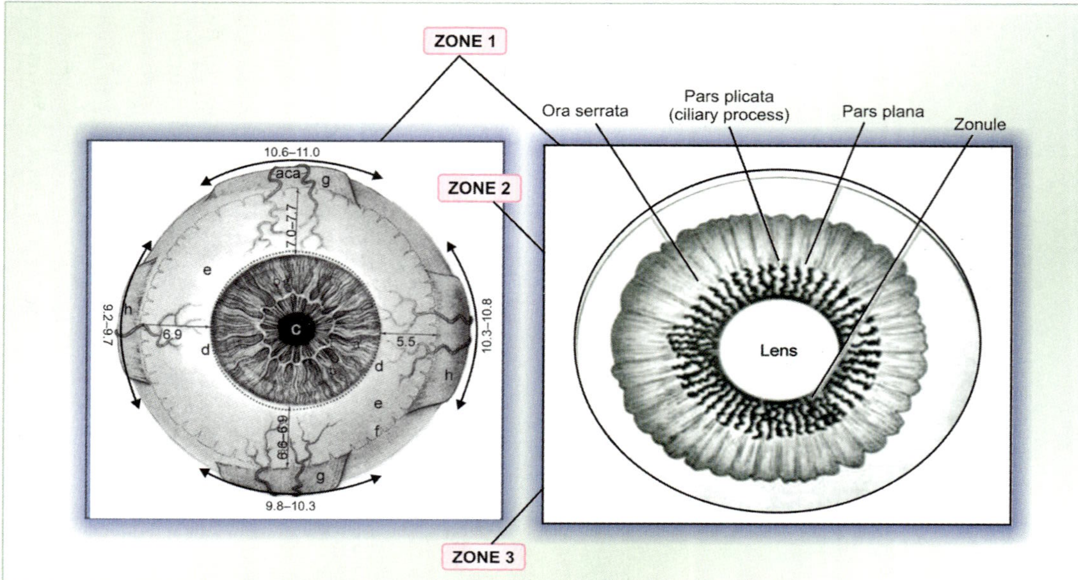

Fig. 16.9: LaserACE™ critical zones—anatomy and geometry

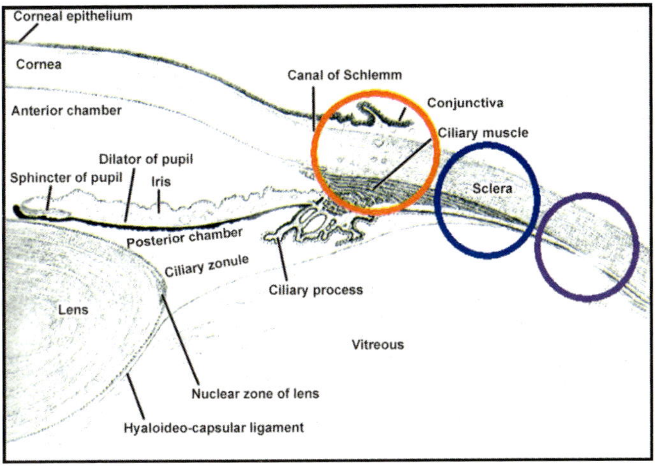

Fig. 16.10: LaserACE™ critical zones—physiology

excisions are made in segmental zones with relativity to the natural physiological shape of the sclera and in tangential quadrants which allows decompression of the functional structures in the physiological planes of the spheroid of the eye globe in three critical zones of anatomical and physiological significance (Fig. 16.10).

Critical Zones

- Zone 1: Just distal to the corneal-scleral envelope in the region of the limbus extending to the pars plana over the girth of the ciliary body/process/complex and particularly the scleral spur 0.5 mm limbal area/tm/scleral spur/structures of the angle.
- Zone 2: The region of the scleral which is begins just outside of pars plana and represents the largest

circumferential diameter of the anterior globe sphere between the equator and the edge of the pars plana.

- Zone 3: The region of the ora serrata and the origin of the anterior radial ciliary muscles.

LASERACE™ NATURAL VISION RESTORATION SURGICAL SOLUTIONS

VisioLite™ Ophthalmic Laser System

The LaserACE™ procedure (Laser Anterior Ciliary Excision) is a revolutionary new technique which is performed with the VisioLite™ Er:YAG laser (Fig. 16.11). The VisioLite™ laser's superior design and ability to control the variations of energy delivered will

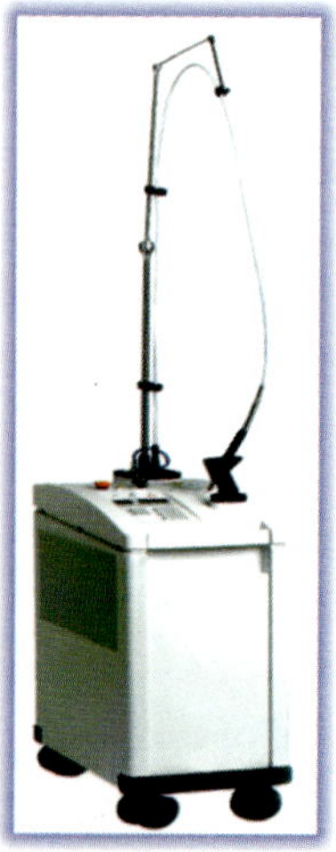

Fig. 16.11: VisioLite™ ophthalmic laser system

be the safest laser on the market for low energy soft tissue ablations for microsurgery in the eye. The laser beam of the VisioLite™ is pulsed and at a specific wavelength (2.94 μm) that is very highly absorbed by water, as well as anything containing water such as CT. The laser beam causes rapid vaporization, or ablation, in both hard and soft tissues. The efficiency of tissue removal varies with the available laser beam wavelength, the energy per pulse, the diameter of the pulse at the target, the pulse duration, and the repetition rate of the pulses. The optimum wavelength for energy absorption in water is 2.94 microns which is what the VisioLite™ ophthalmic laser system emits. The laser energy causes a vaporization of the water in the target tissue, causing an expansion of the water volume. The expansion causes the surrounding mineral material to be ejected. This water mediated explosive tissue

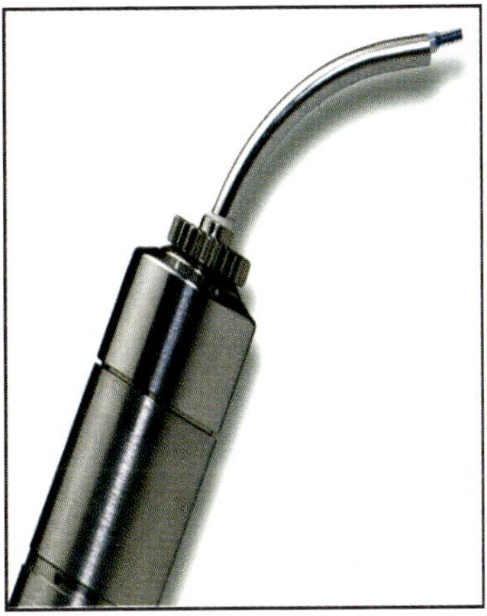

Fig. 16.12A: VisioLite patented optical probe and tip

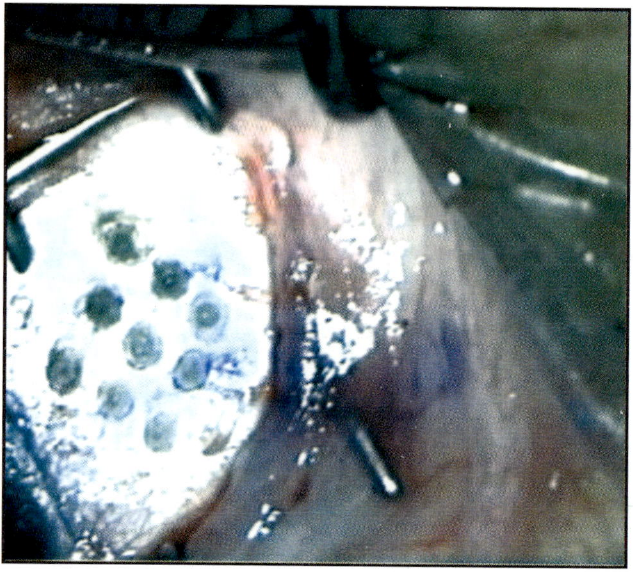

Fig. 16.12B: LaserACE^{TM} NeoPores *in vivo*

removal is efficient and *transfers minimal heat to the surrounding tissue.* The unique properties of the Er:YAG laser allow inhibition of tissue healing response therefore preserving the "NeoPores" integrity without tissue regeneration or scarring. In addition to the Er:YAG being the ideal wavelength to create efficient photoablation without significant photocoagulation[44] (Figs 16.12B and C). There are small 'desirable' thermal and mechanical effects that produce stimulation of proprioceptive and vascular tissues in the ciliary complex which facilitate accommodation. It is further proposed that the unique characteristics of the 2.94 Er:

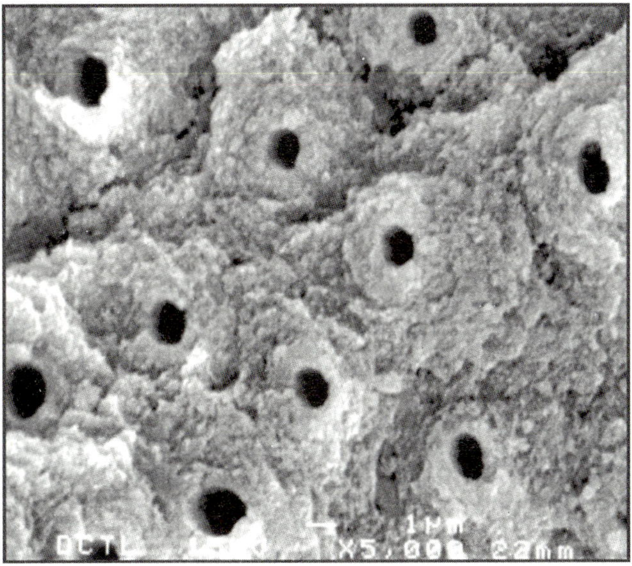

Fig. 16.12C: LaserACE^{TM} NeoPores (SEM 5,000 X)

YAG laser especially contribute to the 'lasting effects' of the procedure by limiting inflammatory stress and inhibiting tissue remodeling.

How LaserACE Works

- *Excisions in the sclera and globe in critical zones thereby restoring the efficiency to the biomechanics of the accommodative system*
- *Secondary impact of changing the biomechanics of the relationship of the lens/ciliary oculociliary joint complex mechanism improves mobility to achieve improved accommodative power.*

- *Improves the efficiency of the hydrodynamic system by influencing intraocular pressure and aqueous drainage. Rejuvenation of the trabecular meshwork.*

LaserACE™: Surgical Technique

The aim of the LaserACE™ surgical procedure is the strategic volumetric decompression of scleral tissue outside the limbus over critical zones of the anterior segment of the globe of the eye. The mathematical model for scleral decompression is based on age-related geometric and tissue characteristics. The scleral decompression is accomplished by removing strategic areas of sclera in opposing quadrants of the anterior globe segment whereby a series of zonal connective tissue partitions are created using a non-contact Er: YAG 2.94 μm wavelength.

The patient is prepared with 2 percent xylocaine topical drops or subconjunctival anesthesia and draped in usual way as LASIK. One percent povidone-iodine is used to prep lashes and cul-de-sac. Mark 6 o'clock and 12 o'clock meridians with a 26 gauge needle dipped in gentian violet an opaque "Hover" contact lens is used with Goniosol or other viscoelastic for corneal protection (Fig. 16.13A). The Critical Zones are mapped out utilizing custom designed quadrant and matrix markers in the 4 oblique quadrants (Figs 16.13B and C). The surgeon determines method of conjunctival dissection either via flap and conjunctival spreader instrument or transconjunctival excision (Fig. 16.13D).

Ideal Eligibility for LaserACE™
Ideal age: 48-65 years
Health patient with no CT diseases or ocular pathology • ±.50 spherical equivalent BCVA 20/25 or better • No more than .50 cylinder • Preferably plano or –.25 to –.50 spherical equivalent prior to LaserACE™ • PRK,RK, LASIK refractive correction can be done either before or after LaserACE™ • Ideally no more than .50 diopters of difference between manifest and cycloplegic refraction
Ideal IOP is 12-20 mm Hg
Normal stereopsis
• No convergence insufficiency or eye teaming deficit, history of fusional problems (phorias and tropias—poor stereopsis) • No excessively large pupils

Calipers are used to measure the total length × width parameters of the exicision zone and a gentian violet marker is used to make outer limit guidemarks for the matrix (Figs 16.14A and B).The VisioLite™ laser and patented optical proble/tip is used to create the "NeoPore" excision matrix. Depending on the protocol used, between 9 to 12 NeoPores are created per quadrant or between 10 to 12 mm cubic volume of sclerotic sclera is removed. The NeoPore depth is approximately 90 to 95 percent (Fig. 16.14C). The resulting "NeoPores" or 'new pores' can be created in a number of design patterns, however, they must have a critical width

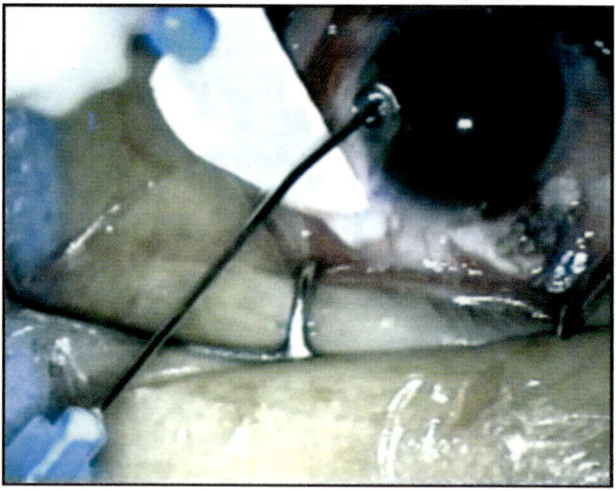

Fig. 16.13A: Preparation for quadrant excisions: Viscoelastic and opaque corneal protector Hover lens with topical anesthetic solution

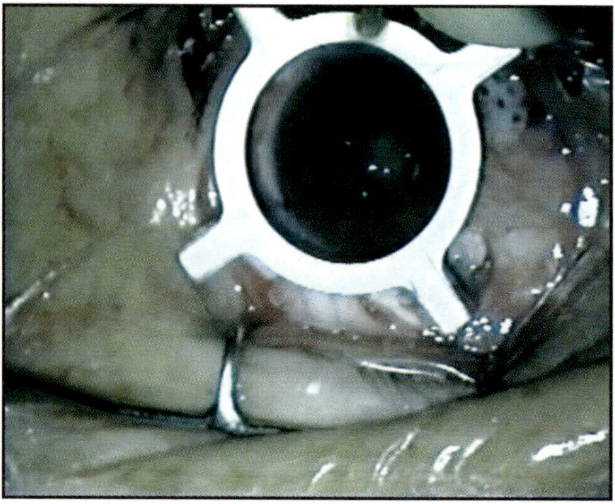

Fig. 16.13B: Four point quadrant marker demarcates central segmental guidelines for "NeoPore" matrix

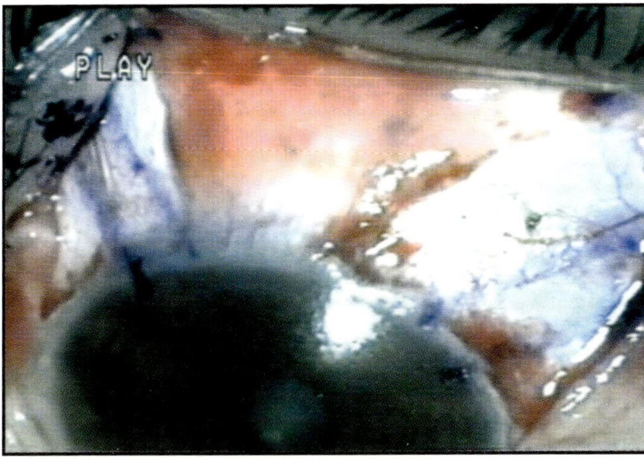

Fig. 16.13C: Conjunctiva is opened to expose parameters of the quadrant zones. Zonal guide marks are used for excision matrix pattern

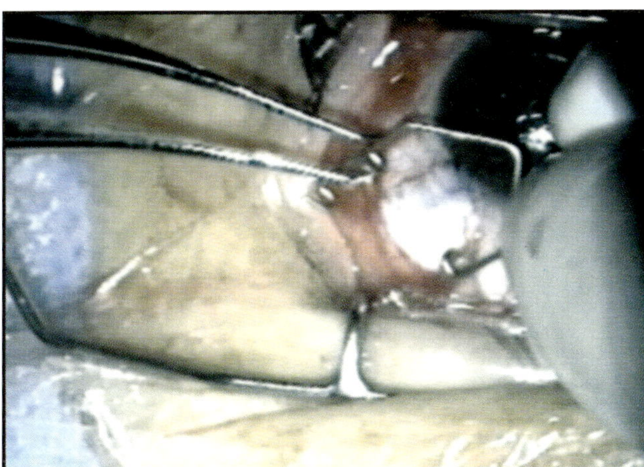

Fig. 16.13D: Conjunctival spreader is used for optimal surgical field

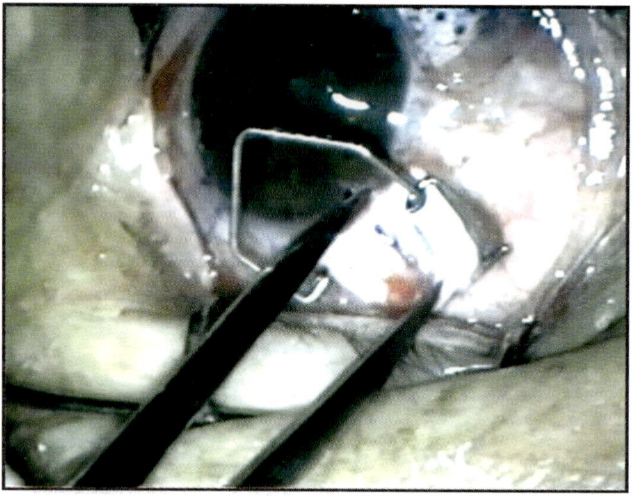

Fig. 16.14A: Calipers are used to measure the total length of the excision zone extending from zone 1-3

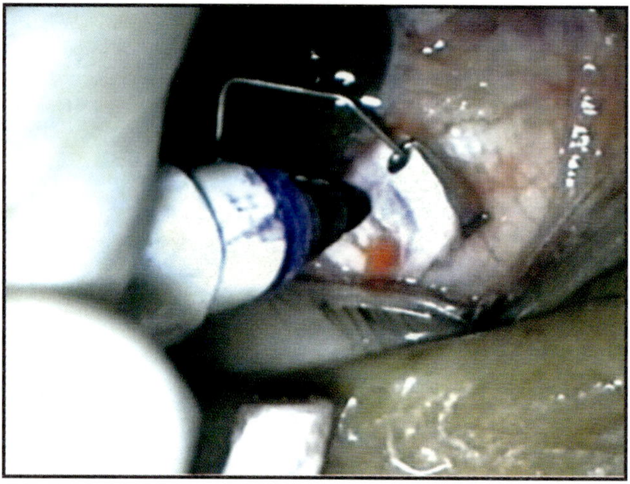

Fig. 16.14B: Excision length and total excision surface area are marked

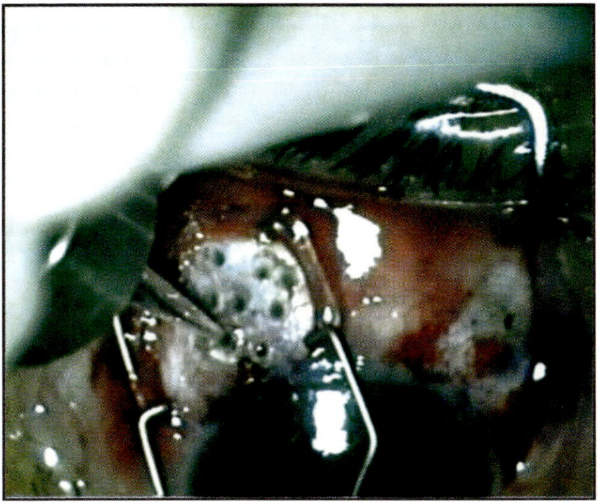

Fig. 16.14C: LaserACE^{TM} "NeoPore" excision matrix is made with the VisioLite patented optical probe tip

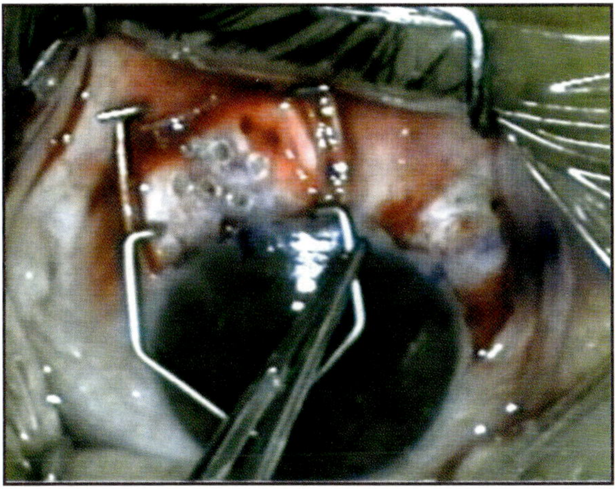

Fig. 16.14D: Completed segmental decompression of sclera is stabilized with opaque bioscaffold fill

which is necessary to inhibit scleral residual tissue approximation thereby inhibiting normal fibroblast activity retarding the connective tissue healing cycle. Collagen reorganization and tissue healing response is further prevented by implantation of a weightless bioscaffold material having very low specific gravity and therefore adding no external loading of the structures beneath and maintaining 'NeoPore' effectiveness (Fig. 16.14D). It is believed that this strategic removal of scleral tissue creates a newly formed microperforated tissue layer at the aponeurosis of the oculus or the subchoroidal lamina within the segmental zone treatment areas. These segmental regions act as biological "flexible diaphragm pumps" or extensible dividing membrane partitions which allow decompression of scleral load and shear stress, rejuvenation of intracellular/extracellular fluid exchange and restoration of biomechanical efficiency in the tissues that are internal to the scleral shell.

The conjunctival spreader is removed after each zone is completed and the conjunctiva is closed with conjunctival glue or alternatively bipolar cautery can be used. Topical anesthetic and steroid drops are placed in the eye following the procedure and are used for one week postoperatively along with biotears. Patient is instructed in VisioFlex™ accommodative exercises immediately.

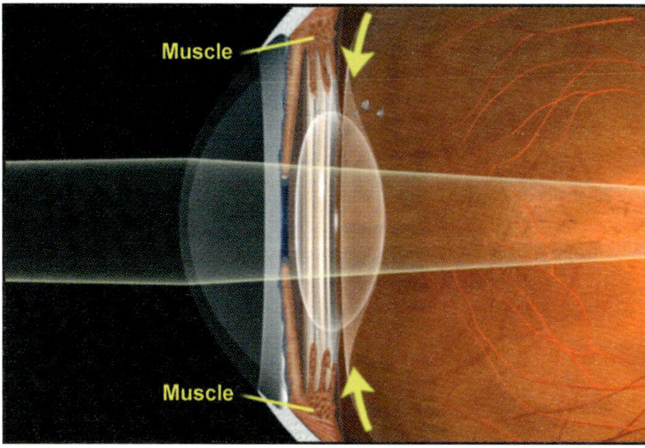

Fig. 16.15: Improved VisioDynamic efficiency with natural restoration of accommodative function

LaserACE^{TM}: Kinesiology Application

The resultant effect of the LaserACE^{TM} procedure is the immediate change in ocular mobility and indirect impact on viscoelastic modulus and rigidity. Enhanced mechanical efficiency of the accommodative mechanism as well as improved aqueous outflow as a result of zonal scleral excisions is demonstrated by an immediate drop in IOP (approximately 3 mm Hg) and ability to respond to near visual stimulus with significant amplitude within a few hours postoperatively. Further implications regarding enhanced metabolic solute transfer in the hydrodynamic system are being studied. It is believed that the culmination of the LaserACE^{TM} decompression results may represent an additional potential prophylactic benefit by producing an improvement of overall eye health and adding the potential effects of increasing the longevity of eye function for satisfactory performance of functional vision ADL with delay of onset of diseased states.

The neuromuscular consequences include a resetting of the oculociliary joint complex in the anterior and posterior chamber, facilitation of the inner scleral wall mobility and choroidal elastic translation of the ciliary ring forces to the lens.[45] The restored biomechanical efficiency may in fact create a positive shift in the AC/C ratio (accommodation convergence/convergence) decreasing the level of effort needed to accommodate.[46] Lens factors still contribute to the overall accommodative deficits but despite this even small changes in vector force translations to the lens produce large functional improvements biomechanical improvements and therefore large functional improvements.[47] This is due to the mass and specific gravity of the lens, compared to mass and specific gravity of the sclera in an aged eye and the postoperative resetting of the ciliary ring lens complex. Even as little as 0.25 mm of anterior translation can contribute a significant change in dioptric power for near response. In addition, the increase in specific gravity and central cortex nuclear mass of the lens which accompanies age actually becomes an advantageous mechanical property to allow for an even greater fulcrum with very low requirement in overall force from the ciliary ring in order to move the lens forward to facilitate near vision acuity. Intermediate vision likewise is dramatically improved.

LaserACE™ patient's also experience "overload" to the accommodative mechanism even at rest due to the restoration of functional capacity of the neuromuscular unit until the initial healing phase begins to stabilize and balance the globe. The "NeoPores" remain completely open for approximately 4 to 6 hours. A thin layer of epithelial cells begin to form in the early healing phase to close the inner fascial layer of the sphere. During this temporary initial phase, over convergence or "super vision" will occur in for a time period prior to acute stability of the healing anterior globe segment (approx. 10-14 days). This is followed by smaller variations in fluctuation, manifest stability (approx. 6-8 weeks), and finally a CNS established end point resting tonus in the accommodative system (approx. 3-6 months). It is critically important during all phases, especially the initial phase for the patient to be compliant in accommodative training exercises in order to maximize potential outcomes. Patients can experience 'overload' and ciliary spasm during prolonged exercise or reading activities especially in the first one or two postoperative months. As the system becomes well trained, accommodative spasm dissipates. It is also imperative for the patient to train the newly activated neuromuscular system in both dynamic burst response and prolonged endurance modes. Accommodative insufficiency is seen more in the myopic eye and underdeveloped neuromuscular systems, whereas accommodative spasm is seen more frequently in hyperopic eye type and well-developed accommodative systems. Semi-permanent/permanent stabilization seems to occur at about 6 months postoperative. Safety and preliminary efficacy have been determined by animal studies and *in vivo* treatment of more than 60 human eyes.

LaserACE™ Prospective Clinical Trial: Preliminary Results

In June 2003, clinical surgical validation of the LaserACE™ procedure along with diagnostic proofs for the VisioDynamic theory were initiated in Moscow Russia, with Dr Dimitrii Dementiev. A series of aberrometry and evaluative studies were performed as well as evolution of the LaserACE™ nomogram parameters and are ongoing. These early endeavors were pivotal to the efficacy of the volumetric calculations that produce the stable LaserACE™ biomechanical result without compromise of ocular stability or asymmetry. In December 2003, clinical surgical studies began in Juarez, Mexico, with investigator Dr Bobby Maddox. Clinical surgeries were performed during 2004 on 8 eyes or 16 patients. Results were encouraging with a mean of 3.1 diopters of improvement for accommodative amplitude for near and intermediate vision with no statistically significant change in manifest refraction. In May 2005, clinical surgical studies began in Valencia, Venezuela, with Dr Jose Manuel Vargas. LaserACE™ was performed on 3 eyes recently with similar preliminary results.

Health Canada approved the LaserACE™ procedure for investigative study in October 2004. Presently ongoing prospective Clinical Trials were initiated with Dr John F Blaylock in British Columbia, Canada. Clinical surgeries were performed during 2004 and 2005 on 20 eyes. The preliminary results represented herein. Patient data demonstrated a good effect in improving near vision and an excellent effect at improving intermediate or "functional" vision. Mean increase for these patients of more than 3.0 diopters. These results include 6 months data for most of the 10 patients, but a minimum of 3 months follow-up on all 10 patients. T test and linear regression analysis were

LaserACE™

Preoperative and Postoperative Exam

- Medical history
- Visual function questionnaire
- Complete eye examination
- Dilated fundus exam
- Video keratography
- Contrast sensitivity
- Manifest and cycloplegic refraction
- Pupillary size
- IOP
- Gonioscopy
- Amplitude of accommodation
- (push-up method)
- Near vision at 35 cm (14")
- Intermediate vision at 60 cm (24")
- Axial length and AC depth
  (Humphrey Zeiss IOL Master)
  Pachymetry

performed and *accommodative amplitude* measured with a 'push-up' and 'pull-up' method utilizing the K-range measurement modified prince rule showed significant increase in accommodative amplitude. Monocular increased by 1.89 ± 1.16 D; (mean ± SD, P= 0.000); Range: –0.1 to +3.8 D and binocular increased by 3.27 ± 2.38 D; (mean ± SD, P = 0.002); Range: 0.2 to +7.6 D.

LaserACE™ resulted in significant improvement of both monocular and binocular near uncorrected visual acuity measured at 40 cm (Fig. 16.16). Even greater improvements were seen for intermediate visual acuity measured at 60 cm (Fig. 16.17). A majority of the patients reported on the patient questionnaire more

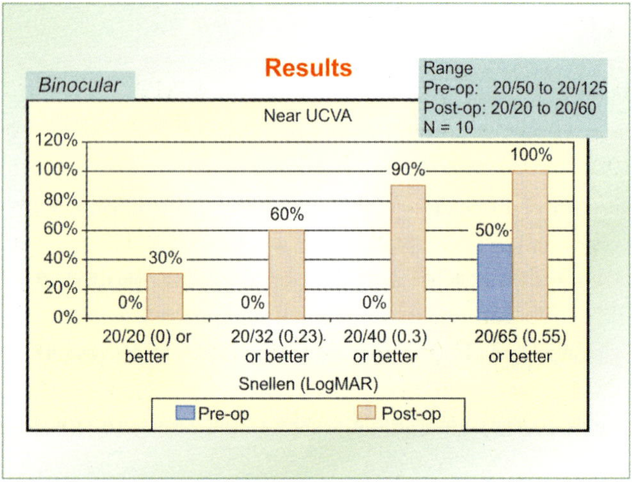

Fig. 16.16: Binocular near uncorrected VA (40 cm) showed significant improvement by 0.47 ± 0.27 (log MAR, mean ± SD) (P = 0.000); Range: 0.17 to 0.90

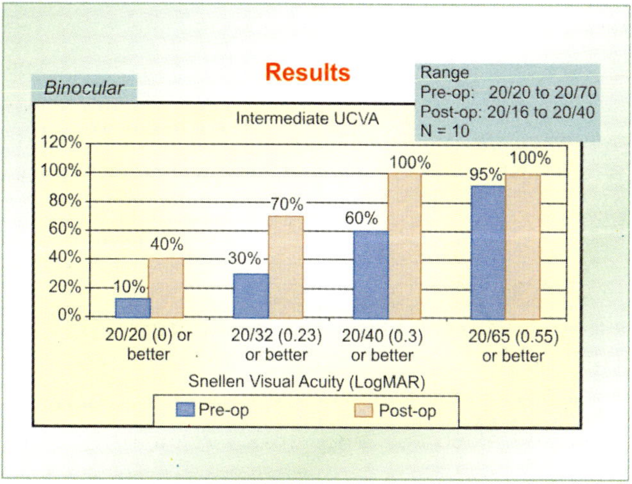

Fig. 16.17: Binocular intermediated uncorrected VA (60 cm) showed improvement by 0.21 ± 0.18 (log MAR, mean ± SD) (P = 0.006); Range: 0.00 to 0.53

dissatisfaction and loss of functional ADL (Activities of Daily Living) with loss of intermediate vision or 'functional-arm's length vision'. Therefore, patient satisfaction for functional ADL was over 95 percent.

LaserACE^{TM} results showed a statistically significant reduction for add diopters for 20/20 of near VA (40 cm) after surgery. Monocular add was reduced by 0.68 ± 0.45 D (mean ± SD) (P=0.000); Range: 0.00 to 1.25 D. Binocular add was reduced by 0.73 ± 0.53 D (mean ± SD) (P=0.002); Range: 0.25 to 1.75 D (Fig. 16.18).

There were minor changes of manifest refraction after surgery, but no statistically significant (P > 0.05);

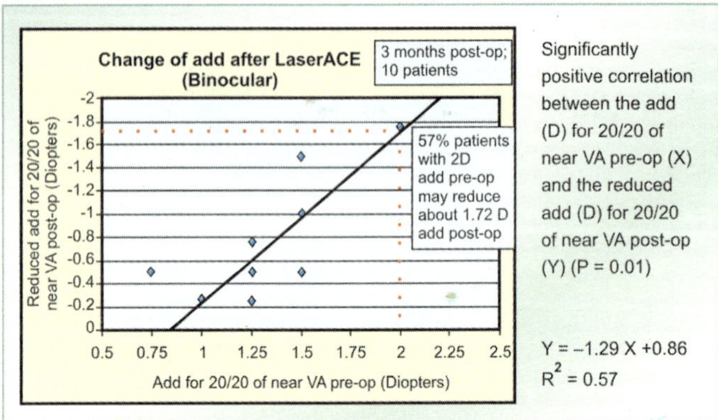

Fig. 16.18: LaserACE™ statistical correlation between add of near VA

Preoperative spherical refraction equivalent; 0.33 ± 0.31 D (mean ± SD); (Range: –0.25 to +0.75 D). Postoperative spherical refraction equivalent 0.31 ± 0.48 D (mean± SD); (Range: –0.50 to + 1.50 D). No statistically significant change of binocular distance uncorrected visual acuity (UCVA); Preoperative UCVA range: 20/15 to 20/25; Postoperative UCVA range: 20/15 to 20/20; N= 10 patients. There were minor changes of manifest refraction after surgery, but no statistically significant (P > 0.05). Preoperative spherical refraction equivalent 0.33 ± 0.31 D (mean ± SD); (Range: –0.25 to +0.75 D); Postoperative spherical refraction equivalent ± 0.48 D (mean± SD); (Range: –0.50 to + 1.50 D). A-scan showed no statistically significant change of axial length (AL) after surgery (P>0.05). Preoperative AL:

Contrast sensitivity

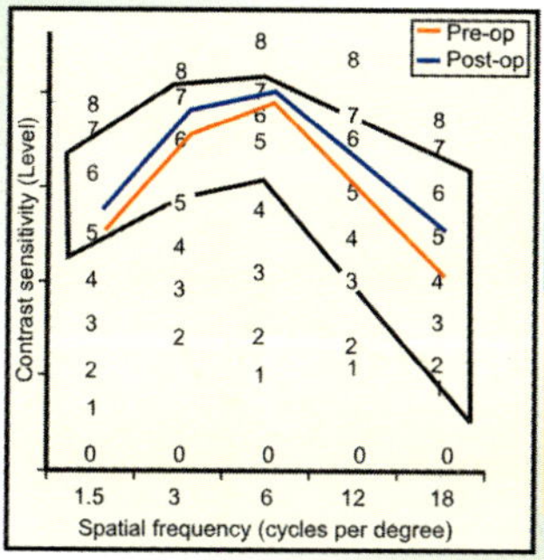

Mean contrast sensitivity level at 5 spatial frequencies before and 3 months after LaserACE

Spatial frequency (cycles per degree)	Mean contrast Sensitivity Level ± SD		P Value
	Pre-op	Post-op	
1.5	5.0 ± 0.6	5.4 ± 0.7	0.06
3	6.1 ± 0.8	6.6 ± 0.9	0.04
6	6.2 ± 1.1	6.8 ± 1.0	0.05
12	4.9 ± 1.0	5.5 ± 1.3	0.06
18	4.0 ± 1.2	5.1 ± 1.6	0.01

Paired samples T test

Fig. 16.19: LaserACE™ statistical correlation between mean contrast sensitivity

23.57 ± 0.97 mm (mean ± SD). Postoperative AL: 23.56 ± 0.98 mm (mean ± SD). Topography (Humphrey) showed no statistically significant change of corneal curvature after surgery ($P > 0.05$). Preoperative average K value: 42.92 ±1.57 D; (mean ± SD); Postoperative average K value: 43.12 ± 1.72 D (mean ± SD).

Early outcomes have also shown a small statistically significant improvement in contrast sensitivity (Fig. 16.19). Review of preoperative patient questionnaire shows that patient compliance with accommodative exercises gives better outcomes as well as patients who read frequently. In patients with previous LASIK or PRK, LaserACE™ appears to be preferred choice for presbyopic solution. Presbyopia with high reading add obtain greater improvement after surgery. Overall preliminary results are promising.

LaserACE™ Complications

Very minor or low complication rate has been reported with the LaserACE™ procedure. No anterior segment ischemia has been reported and no major complications. Patients experience temporary ciliary fimosis initially which can be alleviated by over the counter pain medications. Temporary redness and dryness is alleviated with biotears. Patients have improvement of near and intermediate vision within hours of the procedure.

LaserACE™
Complications

- Two conjunctival cysts
- No ASI
- Subconjunctival hemorrhage
- No dry eye problem
- Temporary redness, and mild to moderate discomfort
- One patient saw shadowing at intermediate VA test in left eye 1 day postoperative and it disappeared within 1 week
- One patient had focusing problem at 20-40 feet 2 weeks postoperative and this disappeared one month postoperative

REFERENCES

1. Hipsley AM. VisioDynamics manuscript. VisioDynamic theory: A biomechanical model for the aging ocular organ 2003.
2. Amile D, Woo SL-Y, Harwood FL, Akeson WH. The effect of immobilization on collagen turnover in connective tissue.

A biochemical-biomechanical correlation. Acta Orthop Scand 1982;53:325.

3. Viidik A, Danielsen CC, Oxluind H. Fourth International Congress of Biorheology Symposium on Mechanical Properties of Living Tissues: On fundamental and phenomenological models, structure and mechanical properties of collagen, elastic and glycosaminoglycan complexes. Biorheology 1982;19:437.
4. Sylvie Wendling A1, Patrick CaÑadas , Christian Oddou A1, Alain Meunier A3. Inter-relations between Elastic Energy and Strain in a Tensegrity Model: Contribution to the Analysis of the Mechanical Response in Living Cells. Computer Methods in Biomechanics and Biomedical Engineering 2002;5(1):1-6.
5. Diamant J, et al. Collagen: Ultrastructure and its relations to mechanical properties as a function of ageing. Proc R Soc Lond (Bio J) 1972;180:293.
6. Dale WC. A composite materials analysis of the structure, mechanical properties, and aging of collagenous tissues. PhD thesis, Case Wetern Reserve University, Cleveland, Ohio 1974.
7. Curtin BJ. "Physiopathological Aspects of Scleral Stress-strain". Tr Am Opht Soc 1969;67:417-61.
8. Fung YCB. Stress-strain history relations of soft tissues in simpole elongation. In Fung YV, Perrone N, Anliker M (Eds). Biomechanics: Its Foundations and Objectives. Englewood Cliffs: Prentice-Hall 1972;1818-208.
9. Werner L, et al. Correlation between different measurements within the eye relative to phakic intraocular lens implantation. J Cataract Refract Surg 2004;30:1982-88.
10. Fung YCB. Biomechanics: Mechanical Properties of Living Tissues. New York: Springer Verlag 1981;222.
11. Hutton RS. Neuromuscular physiology. In Welsh RP, Shephard RJ (Eds): Current Therapy in Sports Medicine. Philadelphia: BC Decker. 1985;1985-86.
12. Aura O, Komi PV. Effects of prestretch intensity on mechanical efficiency of positive work and on elastic behaviour of skeletal muscle in stretch-short cycle. Int J Sports Med 1986b;7:137.

13. Craik R. Biomechanics: A neural control perspective. Physical Therapy 1984;64:1810-11.
14. Hipsley AM. VisioDynamics Manuscript: Biomechanical Solutions for the Aging Ocular Organ: LaserACE^{TM} Natural Vision Restoration.
15. Arciniegas A, Amaya LE. Mechanical behavior of the sclera. Ophthalmologica 1986;193(1-2):45-55.
16. Paul JP. Approaches to design: Force actions transmitted by joints in the human body. Proc R Soc Lond B 1976; 192,163.
17. Sigal IA, Flanagan JG, Tertinegg I, Ethier RC. Finite Element Modeling of Optic Nerve Head Biomechanics. Investigative Ophthalmology and Visual Science. 2004;45: 4378-87.
18. Ioannis G Pallikaris, 1,2 George D Kymionis,1,2 Harilaos S. Ginis, 2 George A. Kounis, 2 Miltiadis K. Tsilimbaris1,2. Ocular rigidity in living human eyes. Invest Ophthalmol Vis Sci 2005;46:409-14.
20. Burgoyne CF, Downs JC, Bellezza AJ, Suh JK, Hart RT. The optic nerve head as a biomechanical structure: A new paradigm for understanding the role of IOP-related stress and strain in the pathophysiology of glaucomatous optic nerve head damage. Prog Retin Eye Res 2005;24(1):39-73.
21. Battaglioli JL, Kamm RD. Measurements of the compressive properties of scleral tissue IOVS: 1984.
22. Rada JA, Achen VR, Penugonda S, Schmidt RW, Mount BA. Proteoglycan composition in the human sclera during growth and aging. Invest Ophthalmol Vis Sci 2000; 41(7):1639-48.
23. Rada JA, Achen VR, Rada KG. Proteoglycan turnover in the sclera of normal and experimentally myopic chick eyes. Invest Ophthalmol Vis Sci 1998;39(11):1990-2002.
24. Yamaoka A, Matsuo T, Shiraga F, Ohtsuki H. TIMP-1 production by human scleral fibroblast decreases in response to cyclic mechanical stretching. Opthalmic Res 2001;3(2):98-101.
25. Watson PG, Young, RD. Scleral structure, organisation and disease: a review. Exp Eye Res 2004;78(3):609-23.

26. Julie Albona, Peter P Purslowb, Wojciech SS Karwatowskic, David L Eastyd. Age-related compliance of the lamina cribrosa in human eyes. Br J Ophthalmol 2000;84:318-23.
27. Gong H, Freddo TF, Johnson M. Age-related changes of sulfated proteoglycans in the normal human trabecular meshwork. Exp Eye Res 1992;55(5):691-709.
28. Koretz JF, Rogot A, Kaufman PL. Physiological strategies for emmetropia. Trans Am Ophthalmol Soc 1995;93:105-18; discussion 118-22.
29. Hanna KD, et al. "Computer Simulation of Arcuate and Radial Incisions Involving the Corneoscleral Limbus", Eye 1989;3:227-39.
30. Ross C Ethier, Mark Johnson, Jeff Rubert. Ocular biomechanics and biotransport. Annual Review of Biomedical Engineering 2004;6:249-73.
31. Neacsu A, Tuchila G, Trifu M, Curea M, Boeru G. Biomechanical stress in glaucoma—cause and effect. Oftalmologia 2004;48(4):93-98.
32. Mori F, Konno S, Hikichi T, Yamaguchi Y, Ishiko S, Yoshida A. Factors affecting pulsatile ocular blood dlow. Br J Ophthalmol 2001;85:529-30.
33. Shepherd RJ. Physiology and Biochemistry of Exercise. Praeger, New York 1982.
34. Buckwalter JA. Maintaining and restoring mobility in middle and old age: the importance of the soft tissues. Instr Course Lect 1997;46:459-69.
35. Norton TT, Siegwart JT Jr. Animal models of emmetropization: matching axial length to the focal plane. J Am Optom Assoc 1995;66(7):405-14.
36. Woo SL-Y, et al. Nonlinear Material Properties of Intact Cornea and Sclera. Exp Eye Res 1972;14:29-39.
37. Robin JB. Radial keratotomy: Procedures. Indian J Ophthalmol 1990;8(3):103-06.
38. Thornton S. Anterior Ciliary Sclerotomy (ACS), A Procedure to Reverse Presbyopia. In Neal Sher (Ed): Surgery for Hyperopia and Presbyopia 1997;33-37.

39. Schachar RA. Cause and treatment of presbyopia with a method for increasing the amplitude of accommodation. Ann Ophthalmol 1992;24:445-52.
40. Lin JT, Perasso A, Martinez D. A novel device for presbyopia reversal. Ann Ophthalmol 1999;92.
41. Hipsley AM. Influence of biomechanics on age-related changes of the eye: Clinical implications for refractive surgery. ASCRS 2005.
42. Strenk SA, Semmlow JL, Strenk LM, Munoz P, Gronlund-Jacob J, DeMarco JK. Age-related changes in human ciliary muscle and lens: A magnetic resonance imaging study. Invest. Ophthalmol Vis Sci 1999;40:1162-69.
43. Battaglioli JL, Kamm RD. Measurements of the compressive properties of scleral tissue. IOVS: 1984.
44. Becker PC, Olsson NA, Simpson JR. Erbium-doped fiber amplifiers: Fundamentals and technology. San Diego [etc]: Academic Press Aron Rosa 1999.
45. Friberg TR, Lace JW. A comparison of the elastic properties of human choroid and sclera. Exp Eye Res 1988; 47(3):429-36.
46. Mutti DO, Jones LA, Moeschberger ML, Zadnik K. AC/A ratio, age, and refractive error in children. Invest Ophthalmol Vis Sci 2000;41(9):2469-78.
47. van Alphen GW. Choroidal stress and emmetropization. Vision Res 1986;26(5):723-34.

CHAPTER 17

A New System (DTK-Plus) for Thermal Keratoplasty using IR Lasers

JT Lin (USA)
Vivek Kadambi (India)

INTRODUCTION

Corneal reshaping procedures, such as photorefractive keratectomy (PRK) and laser assisted *in situ* keratomileusis (LASIK) have been performed by lasers in the ultraviolet (UV) wavelength of 193 to 213 nm. The commercial UV refractive lasers include ArF excimer laser (at 193 nm) in US Pat. 4,773,414 of L'Esperance, et al and other non-excimer, solid-state lasers such as those proposed by Lin in 1992 (US Pat. No. 5,144,630) and in 1996 (US Pat. No. 5,520,679). The above-described systems using lasers to reshape the corneal surface curvature, however, are limited to the corrections of myopia, hyperopia and astigmatism (Table 17.1). They do not significantly contribute to the treatments of presbyopia or glaucoma.

Refractive surgery using a scanning device and lasers in the mid-infrared (mid-IR) wavelength was first proposed by Lin in US Pat. No. 5,144,630 and 5,520,679 and later proposed by Telfair et al in US Pat. No. 5,782,822. These inventions disclosed the generation of mid-IR wavelength of 2.5 to 3.2 microns, by various methods including, but not limited to, the Er:YAG laser (at 2.94 microns), the Raman-shifted solid-state lasers (at 2.7-3.2 microns) and the optical parametric oscillation (OPO) lasers (at 2.7-3.2 microns).

Hyperopia may be surgically corrected by LASIK which involves corneal tissue removal. Alternatively, minimally invasive techniques may be employed using

Ho:YAG laser (at 2070-2120 nm) or the diode laser (at 1885 nm), through thermal keratoplasty procedures known as Holmium Laser Thermokeratoplasty (Ho: LTK) and Diode Laser Thermokeratoplasty (DTK), respectively. Radiofrequency (RF) wave can also be used to create the same effect by a procedure known as conductive keratoplasty (CK).[1-4] Procedures of LASIK, Ho:LTK, DTK and CK have also been recently used for the correction of presbyopia which is limited to monovision treatment by inducing myopia in the nondominant eye. This is in contrast to the laser scleral ablation (LASA) procedure which normally treats both eyes and does not result in any myopic shift.[5,6]

HYPEROPIA CORRECTION (TABLE 17.2)

The recent paper of Rehany and Landa[3] reported results of DTK using a diode laser having a focusing optics for contact mode with deeper penetration of the laser thermal energy in the corneal stroma. However, their data still showed significant six-month post-operative regression of about 0.7 diopter. Papadopauls et al[2] using non-contact Ho:LTK in 50 hyperopic eyes showed that 32 cases reached refraction stability within 1 to 3 months follow-up, 5 cases within 3 to 6 months and 3 cases within 12 months. Their data also showed a similar regression as that of DTK. The major factor responsible for postoperative regression with Ho:LTK and DTK, is the cone-shaped laser power profile (or temperature profile) within the corneal stroma, where

Table 17.1: Summary of Technologies for Vision Corrections (laser and nonlaser methods)

1.	PRK, LASEK, EPI-LASIK	Corneal surface ablation with laser (epithelium removed or preserved); suitable for low diopter corrections (< 3.5 D) or high diopter with thin cornea; simple procedure.
2.	LASIK	Stroma ablation by laser after a "flap" is prepared by microkeratome; (less pain, fast recovery, epithelium intact, less haze); potential keratome failure, thin cornea, flap complication.
3.	LASA, LACA	Presbyopia treatment by laser scleral ablation (LASA) to increase accommodation via ciliary body contraction; combining effects of change in scleral elasticity, lens curvature change and anterior chamber shift. Efficiency may be improved by deeper laser ciliary-body ablation (LACA)
4.	LZT, LCT	Laser zonules thermal (LZT) stimulation for presbyopia: non-invasive method using gona lens and focused laser. Laser ciliary-body thermal shrinkage (LCT) for presbyopia
5.	SEB	Scleral expansion band implanted in scleral layer to cause near vision improvement; major regression
6.	ACS	Anterior ciliary sclerotomy by diamond knife incision; major regression which may be reduced by silicon expansion plug.

Contd...

Table contd...

7.	CK	Conductive keratoplasty using radio frequency wave for hyperopia and monovision correction; treated eye to see near but losing its far vision; non-surgical, corneal curvature changed via thermal shrinkage
8.	LTK and DTK	Laser thermal keratoplasty (LTK) using Ho:YAG (at 2.1 um) or diode laser (1.45 to 2.1 micron) (DTK)
9.	MFCR	Multi-focal corneal reshaping by excimer LASIK
10.	AIOL	Accommodative IOL implanted to lens capsule; forward movement for accommodation; good for post-cataract eyes; loop, thin plates, human optics
11.	MIOL	Multi-focal IOL implanted for patient with high refraction errors
12.	Super Vision	Customized LASIK combined with wave-front technology; flying-spot scanning laser with eye tracking is required for customized and irregular corneal reshaping

**Major technologies (inventors):* Broad beam Excimer (L'Esperance, Blum, Taboada); LTK (Sand); SEB (Schachar); Flying-spot LASIK (Lin); LAPR and LACA (Lin), LZT (Lin, Martinez); Eye-tracking (Lai); Solid-state UV Laser for LASIK (Lin, Lai); MFCR (Ruitz). Most of the above technologies have been patented (1988-2004) and greater details may be found in their patents by online searching of "US Patent" files or by the following US pat. No: 4718418, 5484432, 5520679, 5144630, 6263879, 6258082, 5533997, 5354331.

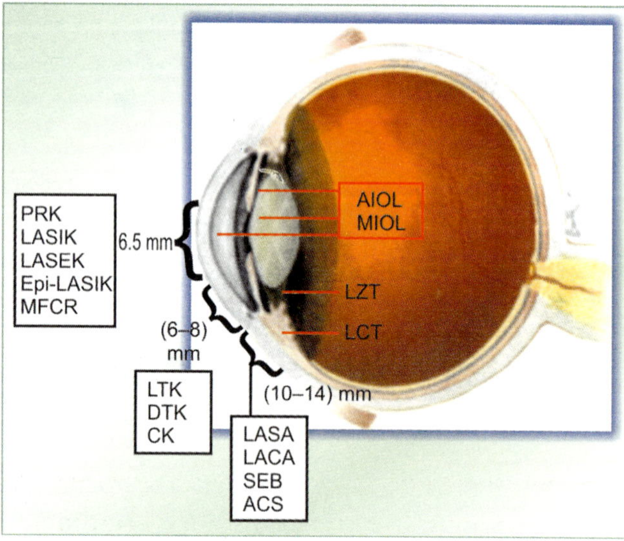

Fig. 17.1: Summary of various technologies for vision correction (referred to Table 17.1 for notations)

the penetration depth (d) is limited by the strong tissue absorption of the laser energy. While the existing DTK system with a tightly focused beam within the stroma may have successfully improved the penetration depth, it did not improve the effective tissue volume (ETV) for collagen shrinkage. The nonfocused Ho:LTK has its majority of laser energy absorbed by superficial stromal layer of about 0.15 mm. To overcome the limitation of penetration depth and maximize the ETV for thermal shrinkage, we propose a new concept based on an optimized focusing beam which was used in a system called DTK-plus by New Vision, Inc. (patent pending).

Table 17.2: Comparison of technologies for hyperopia correction

Method	*Features*
LASIK	ArF excimer laser corneal surface ablation
Ho:LTK	Ho:YAG laser (at 2.1 micron) non-focused beam, shallow penetration
DTK	Diode-laser (at 1.88 micron), focused CW beam
DTK-Plus	Diode-laser (at 1.4-1.9 micron), optimal focused beam
CK	Penetration depth controlled by electrode length

PENETRATION DEPTH

The laser power density profile (or irradiance/transmittance profile) of a focused laser inside an absorbing medium, in this case, ocular tissue, may be calculated by a revised Beer's law:

$$P = B\exp(-dA) \qquad \text{(Eq. 1)}$$

$$B = [f / (f-d)]^2 \qquad \text{(Eq. 2)}$$

where A is the absorption coefficient of the cornea tissue at a given laser spectrum; B is a focusing factor which is inversely proportional to the focused beam spot size (derived from simple geometry); f is the focal length of the optics and d is the penetration depth or position away from the corneal surface, which in case of contact mode equals zero. It should be noted that when d approaches f, B is calculated by the square of the ratio between the initial beam spot size (at d = 0) and the beam waist (a diffraction-limited finite size at d = f) to avoid the singularity of formula (2). From above formula, one may readily see that the laser irradiance has a fast exponential decrease due to its absorption in ocular tissue, which is competing with the increasing factor B in a focused beam. The net result of power absorption and beam spot decrease (or increase of power density) produces a peak value (P*) of the laser irradiance profile located at the focal point or position of minimal beam spot. For example, given a laser spot size (diameter) of 1.0 mm on the corneal surface (or d = 0) which is focused to a minimal spot of 0.25 mm (at d = f), one may easily calculate, from Eq. 2, B = (1, 4, 16, 4, 1) at d/f = (0, 0.5, 1.0, 1.5, 2.0).

Using the published transmittance data (Atchinson and Smith, "Optics of human eye", p. 108) to calculate the absorption coefficient[7] (A) to be about 20 to 70 cm^{-1} for laser wavelength at about 1.4 to 2.1 micron, the absorption term exp(-dA) may be calculated at various penetration depth (d).

Several important features may be addressed based on the above calculated profiles. The peak irradiance (P*) of a focused laser is inversely proportional to the absorption coefficient (A), i.e. a laser having a larger A value has a lower P* than that having a smaller A value. However, this peak power effect from focusing factor (B) may be totally suppressed by the exponentially decreasing term by an appropriate choice of the focal length (f). Mathematically, a perfect flat-top (PFT) profile would be possible under the condition of B = exp (+dA) for all depth (d). For A = 55 cm^{-1} as an example, the PFT condition is given by B = (1.0, 3.96, 7.9, 15.7) at depth position of d = (0, 0.25, 0.375, 0.5) mm. This PFT condition is fundamentally impossible to meet under a typical lens design having B = (1, 4, 7.1, 16) for spot size of (1, 0.5, 0.37, 0.25) R, R being the spot size on the corneal surface which produces an almost flat-top (AFT) oscillating function. These AFT profiles require a deeper focal point (f) at 1.0 mm (or two times of the corneal thickness) for the case of A = 30 cm^{-1}. In general, the condition for AFT profile is given by B* = exp (f*A), therefore, f* = (0.92, 0.7, 0.62, 0.55, 0.46) mm, for A = (30, 40, 45, 55, 60) cm^{-1}.

The laser irradiance profile is almost flat in the vertical (depth), the laser footprint (spot size) is conical in shape in a focused beam. Therefore, no homogeneous laser irradiance profile exists in both vertical and horizontal directions. The most one may achieve is an approximate flat-top (AFT) profile in the depth direction and under the condition defined above. To achieve maximal thermal shrinkage tissue volume (MTTV), the preferred focal length includes:

f = f*+/–0.2 mm for small A = (20 to 35) cm^{-1}, and

f = f*+/–0.05 mm for large A = (40 to 70) cm^{-1}.

TEMPERATURE PROFILE

For RF devices, the penetration depth is controlled by the configuration of the electrode tip. For IR laser of

1.4 to 2.2 microns, the absorption (0.5 mm path) in cornea, sclera or conjunctival tissue is about 60 percent (at 1.4 micron), 75 percent (at 1.45, 1.87 and 2.1 micron), 50 percent (at 1.8 micron), 95 percent (at about 1.89 micron) and over 99 percent (at about 1.92 microns) for non-focused beam.[7] These are the criteria for the selected IR lasers in addition to the focusing factor (B) discussed earlier. The absorption depth at various laser spectra for various ocular tissues is one of the critical elements in defining system parameters of this invention. Given value of "A" with respect to the treated tissue, we may predict the penetration depth (d) by the revised Beer's law, Bexp $(-A \times d)$ discussed earlier. However, the penetration depth is also an increasing function of the power of the thermal energy beam.

As shown earlier, higher "A" values tend to move the temperature peak profile forward towards the corneal epithelium. Therefore, to avoid cornea epithelial damage while achieving significant deep thermal penetration, the laser wavelength and the focal length must be carefully specified.

Figure 17.2 schematically shows the temperature profile of the treated tissue relative to the surface temperature "Ts" based on the calculated laser power density profiles. Figures 17.2A to D, respectively represents temperature profiles for non-focused, short-focused ($f < f^*$), optimally focused (with $f = f^*$) and long focused ($f > f^*$) cases, where f^* is defined by $B^* = \exp$

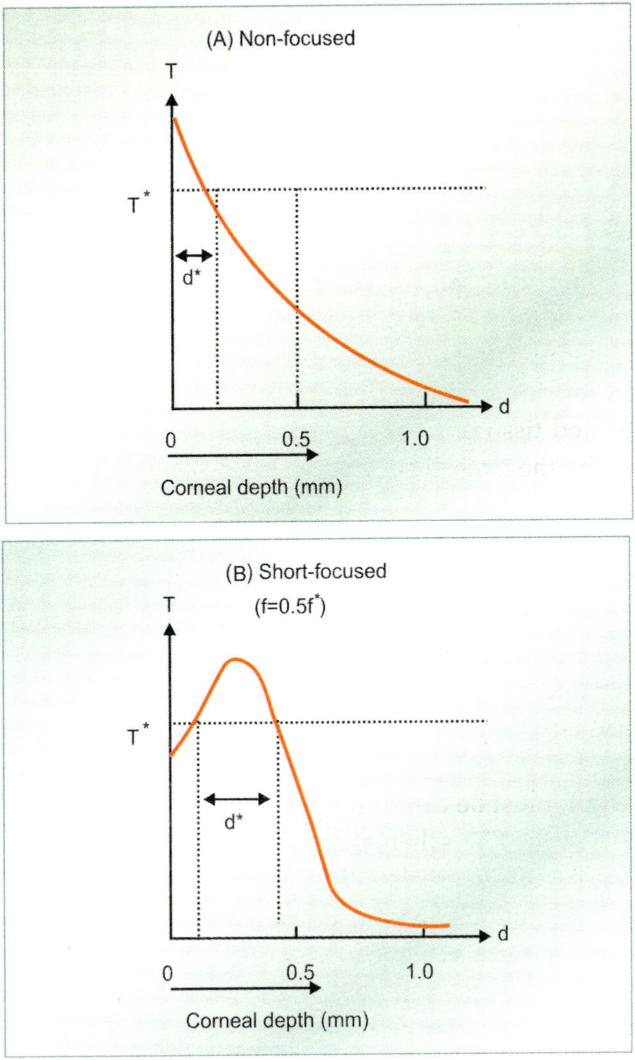

Figs 17.2A and B

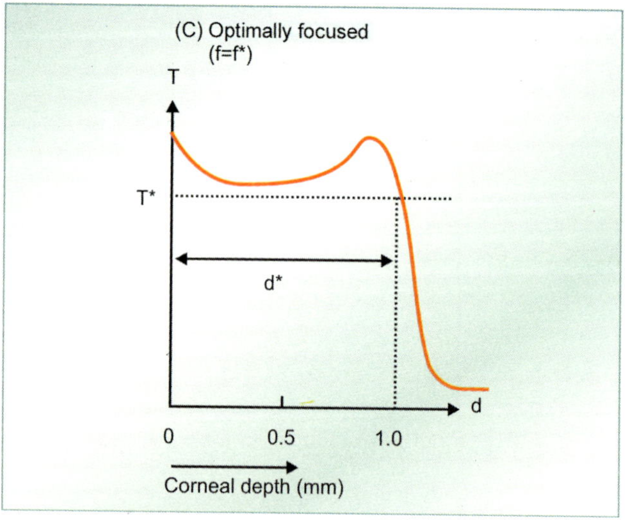

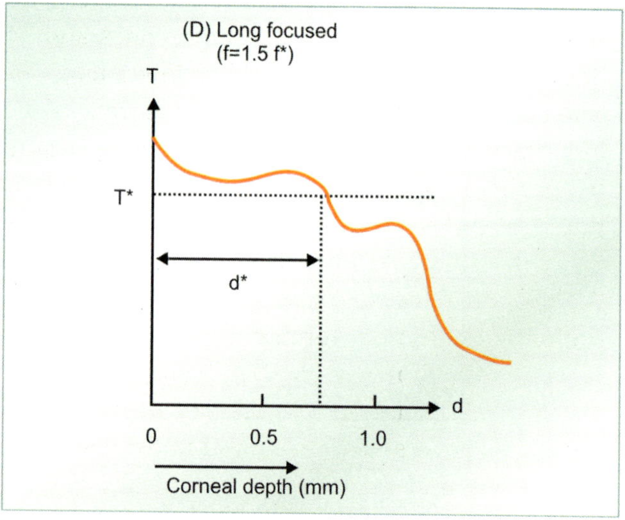

Figs 17.2A to D: Temperature profiles for nonfocused and focused laser, where the Threshold temperature (T*=58°C) defines the penetration depth (d*)

(f*A), or f* = (ln B*/A), and where B* = (7-16) is the value at focal point.

It was known (Stringer HPT, Nature, vol. 204, p.1307, 1964) that stroma collagen shrinkage temperature is 58°C (defined as the threshold temperature "T*") to 75°C. Given the T*, we may evaluate the effective penetration depth (d*), the depth where tissue thermal shrinkage starts to effectively occur. As shown by Figure 17.2 (A) to (D), d* increases with f up to about f = f*, then it starts to decrease after f* and approaches to the non-focused value.

The significance of Figure 17.2 may be summarized as follows:

a. Non-focused laser has the shortest effective penetration, d* = (0.1-0.2) mm depending on A and T*.
b. Short focused case with f < f* has lower temperature on the treated surface, and therefore less risk of surface damage. However, this scenario results in a higher temperature in the vicinity of the endothelial (about 0.5 mm for the case of cornea) and hence the concern of endothelial damage increases.
c. At the optimal focusing case (f = f*), the temperature profile is almost flat-top, similar to that of laser power profile shown in Fig. 17.2, therefore it has the maximal d* whereas the risk of epithelial or endothelial layers may be reduced under controlled laser power and treatment time, typically about 1 to 5 seconds.

d. For long focused beam (f > f*), the value of d* decreases. To keep d* at least 80 percent of the corneal stroma thickness (0.5 mm), as an example, the preferred parameters of this invention includes f is about (0.8-1.5) and most preferable (0.9-1.1) times of f*, where f* is about 0.4 to 1.4 mm, for B* = 16. The preferred range selection of focal length also significantly reduces the risk of overheating on the epithelial or endothelial tissue of the cornea.

SAFETY AND EFFICACY

Non-focused LTK used in Ho:YAG laser (by Sunrise Technologies, Inc.) suffers the disadvantages of shallow penetration, typically less than 1/3 of the cornea stroma thickness. In order to increase the effective penetration depth (d*), defined by the region where stroma temperature is higher than the shrinkage threshold (T*), one needs to use a higher laser power which causes excessive injury to the epithelial layer. Using a focused laser will improve d* and reduce the risk of epithelial damage. However, for short focal length case, used in the conventional DTK system (ProLaser), as shown in Figure 17.2(B), with the focal point inside the stroma increases the risk of endothelial layer damage because of the peak-power profile may be too close to the layer. DTK-Plus system (New Vision, Inc.) using an optimal focal length (f*) about 0.8 to 1.2 mm, longer than the corneal thickness, has a minimal risk of epithelial or endothelial damage, while offering a much deeper d*, in the range of about 0.4 to 0.6 mm.

Conductive keratoplasty (CK) using RF wave electrode may offer a rather deep thermal penetration, controlled by the length of the conductor tip, however, it has been shown to cause scaring and postoperative regression. Regression and poor predictability are the two major drawbacks of existing systems of the CK device, Ho:YAG LTK and conventional DTK. These problems are mainly caused by epithelial or stroma tissue healing and poor control over the temperature profile produced by the thermal energy beam, which may be laser induced or RF wave generated. The conventional-DTK (ProLaser) uses a diode laser at about 1885 nm and having a tolerance of 5 nm which causes the absorption coefficient (A) to change from 40 to 55 cm^{-1}. This uncertainty in A value and the rather long exposure time (about 4 seconds in each treated spot) may result in the change of d* and temperature profile which leads to poor predictability. The new DTK-Plus system (New Vision, Inc.) uses a lower and narrower "A" value at a proprietary wavelength. This not only offers a deeper d*, which is controlled by the optimal local length given by $f^* = (\ln B^*)/A$, with B* about 16, but also repeatable temperature profiles from spot to spot at a shorter exposure time of about 2 to 3 seconds. Therefore, it offers better predictability of refractive outcomes with less regression due to less damage to epithelial or endothelial layer. In addition, a smaller spot size of about 200 micron in DTK-Plus versus about 50 micron in conventional DTK system, reduces the stromal overheating caused by the hot-spot of small laser spot size at the focal point.

Both conventional-DTK and DTK-Plus produce a conical temperature profile, however, DTK-Plus, by virtue of its energy focal length, has a horizontal profile about two times wider than that of conventional DTK. It is important to note that the hyperopic refractive change at a given laser power exposed to the treated spot is proportional to d*W, which is equal to (effective penetration depth) × (mean width of the conical profile). Therefore deeper "d*" and wider width "W" will result in higher diopter hyperopia correction, even when a lower laser power is used. In the CK device, a cylindered temperature profile and deep d* are achievable by the length of conductor tip (about 450 micron). However, a typical tip diameter is only about 90 micron which limits the width (W) of the temperature profile to about 200 micron or less, in comparison to about 200 to 600 micron width in DTK-Plus, and about 50 to 150 micron width in conventional DTK.

The currently used Ho:LTK, DTK devices still suffer instability and postoperative regression which may be significantly reduced by choosing an optimal focusing depth associated to the absorption coefficient (A) at a given laser spectrum.

The threshold temperature (T*) for permanent thermal shrinkage (PTT) of the treated tissue is about

58 degree C. It is important to note that PTT occurs near the surface layer of the treated area in a collimated beam, whereas it penetrates deeply into the area defined by the focal point (or focal length f) in a focused beam. Deep penetration is one of the critical elements for efficacy and postoperative stability presented in this new system. The Ho:LTK system of Sand suffers major regression due to its noncontact, nonfocused superficial laser heating. The new system of DTK-Plus in focused mode overcomes the drawback of prior systems and also provides other advantages including less damage to the corneal epithelial and endothelial layers. It creates sufficient coagulation in almost the entire stroma versus only less than 30 percent in non-focused cases. The prior system of Sunrise Technologies using a non-focused short pulsed Ho: YAG laser results in epithelial damage since the laser power peaks on the surface and causes insufficient coagulation in deep stroma. The currently used conventional DTK using tightly focused CW diode laser (with f about 0.3 to 0.5 mm) improves the penetration depth, however, it still has a narrow peak profile which results in post-operative regression and a low initial efficacy, of less than 2.0 diopter of correction. The broader laser profile under the AFT condition introduced in this chapter not only provides better efficacy for higher hyperopic correction of up to +4 diopter, but also reduces the postoperative regression.

CONCLUSION

Thermal keratoplasty using either CK, non-focused, pulsed Ho:YAG laser (Ho:LTK) or focused CW diode lasers (conventional DTK and DTK-Plus) offer the advantages of being minimally invasive with reduced risk of complication in comparison with LASIK for hyperopia or monovision presbyopia treatment. CK, Ho:LTK and DTK also have the advantage of low system cost. However, the refractive predictability and postoperative regression are the major drawbacks when compared to LASIK. The new DTK-Plus system, with better predictability and higher refractive correction capability than the conventional-DTK and CK, therefore, may be a better alternative for hyperopia correction. Furthermore, a combined procedure (JT Lin, unpublished, pending patent) for thermal shrinkage of corneal stroma and ocular tissues located outside the limbus would have futuristic applications in the treatment of presbyopia.

REFERENCES

1. Alio JL, Ismail MM, Sanchez-Pego JL. Correctional of hyperopia with non-contact Ho:YAG laser thermal keratoplasty. J Refract Surg 1997;13:17-22.
2. Papadopauls NT, Balidis M, Brajitikos PD, et al. Non-contact Ho:YAG laser thermal keratoplasty for hyperopia: two-year follow-up. J Refract Surg 2005; 21:82-86.
3. Rehany U, Landa F. Diode laser thermal keratoplasty to correct hyperopia. J Refract Surg 2004;20:53-61.

4. Pallikaris IG, Nroumidi TL, Pangopoulou SI, Alegakis AK, Astyrakakis NI. Conductive keratoplasty for low moderate hyperopia: 1-year results. J Refract Surg 2003;19:496-506.
5. Lin JT, Mallo O. Treatment of presbyopia by infrared laser radial sclerotomy. J Refract Surg 2003;19:465-67.
6. Lin, JT, Kadambi V. The new mechanism for laser presbyopia reversal and accommodation: Presbyopia, A Surgical Textbook. Thorofare, NJ: Slack Inc; 2002;63-70.
7. Atchison and Smith. Optics of the Human Eye, Butterworth-Heinemann, 2000;110.

Index

H

K

L

M

N

O

P

R

S